THE PILL

ROBERT W. KISTNER, M.D.

the pill

FACTS AND FALLACIES ABOUT TODAY'S ORAL CONTRACEPTIVES

A SEYMOUR LAWRENCE BOOK
DELACORTE PRESS / NEW YORK

*Grateful acknowledgment is made to the following for permission
to quote from material already published:*

American Medical Associates and Victor A. Drill, M.D., Ph.D.
for "Oral Contraceptives and Thrombophlebitis" published in
JAMA, The Journal of the American Medical Association,
September 30, 1968.

J. B. Lippincott Company and Frank Ayd, Jr., M.D. for
"Contraceptives for Teenagers." Reprinted from *Medical Science,*
September 1967, by permission of the authors and publisher.

The National Observer for *The Pill,* a Newsbook.

Prentice-Hall, Inc. and Sherwin A. Kaufman, M.D. for material
from *The Ageless Woman* by Sherwin A. Kaufman.

The Reader's Digest and Grace Naismith for material from
"Common Sense and the Femininity Pill."

Redbook for "The Pill" by Sam Blum. Originally published in
Redbook Magazine, January 1966. Copyright © 1965 by McCall
Corporation.

The chart "U.S. Birthrate Is Near Depression Levels" on page
267 is reprinted from *U.S. News & World Report,* June 24, 1968.
Copyright 1968 U.S. News & World Report, Inc.

Contents

III. THE PILL AND WOMEN'S DISORDERS

IV. PSYCHOLOGICAL, SOCIAL, AND MORAL EFFECTS OF THE PILL

Acknowledgments

No work of this scope could be undertaken, let alone completed, as a personal venture. I cannot possibly name the hundreds of colleagues, students, and patients from whom I have learned so much, but I would like to express my gratitude to: Dr. Arthur T. Hertig, Shattuck Professor of Pathology in the Harvard Medical School, for first stimulating my interest in endometriosis and endometrial cancer—diseases that led me into the field of estrogen-progestin research; Dr. John Rock, Emeritus Clinical Professor of Gynecology in the Harvard Medical School, for guidance during the early days of "Pill" research; Dr. Louis M. Hellman, Professor and Chairman of the Department of Obstetrics and Gynecology in the Downstate New York College of Medicine, and Dr. N. S. Assali, Professor of Obstetrics and Gynecology, University of California at Los Angeles, for sharpening my scientific acuity; Dr. George V. Smith, Emeritus Professor and Chairman of the Department of Gynecology in the Harvard Medical School, for suggesting that I delve into the problem of ovulation; and Drs. Herbert W. Horne, Jr., and Donald G. McKay, whose observations led to the "pseudopregnancy" treatment of endometriosis—my first investigative effort with the Pill.

xii   *Acknowledgments*

I am also indebted to Dr. William J. Crosson for providing me with an adequate supply of an estrogen-progestin combination in 1956 when none was available; to Dr. Victor Drill for his assistance in the initiation of our animal experiments concerning the effects of progestins on endometrial cancer; to Dr. Celso R. Garcia for valuable information regarding the metabolic and long-term effects of estrogen-progestin combinations; to Drs. Paul A. Younge and John F. Jewett for permitting me to utilize their patients in our very early clinical investigations; to Dr. Christopher J. Duncan for his wise counsel and continued moral support.

It would be impossible to express my indebtedness to the hundreds of medical journals, newspapers, magazines, and books consulted over the last decade in preparation for this book. But I would like to pay special tribute to *Ob-Gyn News, Medical Tribune,* and *Medical World News, Redbook, Cosmopolitan, McCall's, Ladies' Home Journal, Saturday Evening Post,* and to Robert Osterman and Mark R. Arnold, authors of *The Pill and Its Impact,* published by the *National Observer.* I have listed references that I thought might be of value to the reader interested in pursuing the subject.

Finally, my sincere appreciation is extended to my secretaries, Mrs. Ann Gregory Metzger, Mrs. Constance Rakoske, Mrs. Linda Angelico, Mrs. Marlene Goldman, and Miss Jean Mackey; to my nurses, Mrs. Dorothy Hislop, Mrs. Nancy Hord, Mrs. Carol Gill, and Mrs. Patricia Arnell; and to Mrs. Harriet Robinson and her staff of nurses in the Outpatient Department of the Gynecologic Division of the Boston Hospital for Women.

"General impressions are never to be trusted. Unfortunately, when they are of long standing, they become fixed rules of life, and assume a prescriptive right not to be questioned. But it is the triumph of scientific men to rise superior to such superstitions, to desire tests by which the value of beliefs may be ascertained, and to feel sufficiently masters of themselves to discard contemptuously whatever may be found untrue."

FRANCIS GALTON

Foreword

THIS IS A BOOK about oral contraceptives, popularly known as "the Pill." Approximately 13 million women around the world use this medication as an aid to family planning. Another million use the same pill for "female disorders"—irregular bleeding, painful periods, and an incapacitating, sterility-producing disease known as endometriosis. These women are a vanguard of about 56 million who, according to present projections, will be taking this compound by 1985.

Why did I write this book? Why should you read it? The answer to both questions is the same. Too little factual information and too much incorrectly interpreted information has flooded every form of news media.

My purpose, therefore, in the preparation of this book was crystal clear. The Pill user sorely needs a reference that provides full and accurate information about the Pill, how it works, its side effects, its complications, its long-term potential. From daily personal contact with thousands of patients taking the Pill under my direction for the last twelve years, I have gained experience, but, more important, I have gained insight into their conflict. Day after day I have noted deep concern, confusion, doubt, fear. Some patients have been ecstatic as a result of their scanty but regular bleeding, an added bonus to pregnancy protection. They had no side effects whatsoever. But others telephoned almost daily about everything—diarrhea, constipation, headaches, leg aches, hand numbness, feet coldness, apathy, jittery nerves, too much libido, too little libido, weight gain, weight loss, hair growth, hair loss. Twenty-five years of experience prescribing medications for the human female helped me not at all. No drug could do all of these things to some patients—and nothing to others. Never before had I looked into defiant and doubting eyes when I made what I believed to be a medically correct statement. "But so-and-so magazine or such-and-such reporter in the whoozis Times says the pills are dangerous. I may die. I might go blind. My next baby may be deformed." How should a physician react to these words? What should he say? The easy road, frequently followed, is to surrender one's conviction to the impact of the headlines, "OK. Skip the pill. Go back to the diaphragm, or condom, or jelly or rhythm, or whatever you wish."

But I have never believed the headlines—nor will I ever sacrifice my own experience to them. An example: About five years ago I gave a paper before the American College of Surgeons on the use of estrogen-progestins during the premenopausal period—a rather dull but exacting report on the effects of the Pill on the lining of the womb. After the formal presentation I was interviewed by the press. Most of the subsequent reports in the newspapers and magazines were factual, but one weekly magazine featured this: "Dr. Robert W. Kistner of Harvard Medical School startled his cohorts at the American College of Surgeons by stating that all women over 40 should be dead." The paragraphs that followed outlined what I really said—but the damage was done.

It is beyond my comprehension to understand how a reporter can detail the "terrible trouble with the Pill" when he has never treated a patient, observed the effects, studied the laboratory data, or tallied the pros and cons. I recall an article describing the permanent effects of the Pill on subsequent suppression of ovulation and resultant infertility. When I later questioned the reporter, I was startled, amazed, and discouraged to note that the writer didn't know what ovulation was, nor how it occurred, nor even

how it was determined. Perhaps this is not his function, but the
reporting of accurate data is.

Perhaps I have attempted to accomplish an impossible task. I
hope not. This is an effort to present all of the facts, and there
are many, in a lucid, concise fashion so that you, the Pill user or
interested reader (possibly both), may weigh the evidence, balance the risks, accept or reject the unproved—then reach your
decision. To project all aspects of the Pill in clear perspective, in
readily understandable prose, is not an easy task. To assist me
in the conversion of mysterious medical terminology to acceptable
language, I have utilized the talents of a gifted writer, Robert A.
Liston. His ability to unmask scientific phrases, to simplify complicated endocrinology, to vitalize the structural formulas of
female hormones has, I hope, distilled my thoughts into readable
sentences.

I am not urging you to take the Pill. I may even convince you not
to take it. But the real purpose of this book is to enable you to
make up your own mind—to provide you with what I believe
to be facts—not fantasy. Then you must make your decision as to
which type of contraception seems most acceptable to you. But
base your decision on factual data—not on fear.

The book is organized to provide at the outset a few basic facts
about the physiology of ovulation, menstruation, and pregnancy.
Without this knowledge it is difficult to understand precisely how
the Pill works. I have included a chapter on other methods of contraception presently available, with comparative risks of pregnancy. Specific female disorders and diseases that may be aggravated or improved by the Pill are discussed simply because
such information is not readily available to the average woman.
Subsequent chapters are designed to explain the causes, prevention, and treatment of the most common side effects and to analyze
critically the short-term and long-term risks. I have tried to place in
proper perspective, from a gynecologist's point of view, the effects
of the Pill on society, teenage mores, the Catholic Church, and the
population explosion.

Finally, let me caution you about reading and interpreting
medical reports. It is difficult even for the experienced investigator

to separate the wheat from the chaff, to know whether a report is of "statistical significance." How can you, a nonmedical person, interpret the data? The answer is, you can't. Try this one: A recent report of a low-income group of patients (in whom the incidence of cancer of the cervix is high) indicated that there was a higher incidence of cervix cancer in Pill users than in diaphragm users. The headlines might read, "Cancer Increased in Pill Users." But, unfortunately, the prevalence of cancer of the cervix in women using neither Pills nor diaphragms was not given. Always look for the "controls," the nontreated group. Actually, a complete study might indicate that the diaphragm protects against cancer of the cervix more than the pill does, but the incidence might be higher in the controls than in the treated patients.

It would be both surprising and depressing if readers were to find nothing to disagree with in my book. Medical science is not static, and I may have to change my mind about issues that now seem clearly settled. Controversy makes the subject exciting. For the moment, this is the way I see it.

R.W.K.

I

CONTRACEPTION

1. A Search for Perspective

THE DEVELOPMENT of oral contraceptives must rank as one of the major achievements of medical science. Popularly known as "the Pill," this medication is one of a very select group of drugs that are virtually 100 per cent effective. It produces only a small number of serious side effects and contraindications are relatively few. As a result, only a minority of women cannot or should not take the Pill. Moreover, this drug is easily manufactured and is sold at a reasonable price. It is simple to take, and the directions for its use are not overly complicated.

Each of these factors is of importance considering the present population crisis. Demographic experts tell us that this planet faces threats of famine, war, and disease if the birth rate is not soon curtailed. Whether or not these fears are exaggerated, the fact remains that any method that is 100 per cent effective in controlling the rate of conception is highly desirable. While the effectiveness of the Pill in controlling the world's birth rate is of primary importance, the Pill has other advantages. Each of these will be discussed in detail in subsequent chapters, but in order to start with a clear perspective about this controversial medication, the advantages and disadvantages should now be considered.

ADVANTAGES

1. Because of its effectiveness, the Pill has enabled millions of couples to achieve family planning. Husbands and wives are now able to have the number of children they desire when they desire them. Since the number of children may be restricted to those who can be properly fed, clothed, housed, and educated, the Pill prevents the tragedy of the unwanted child. When this advantage has been widely acknowledged in underdeveloped but overpopulated countries, the Pill, or a variation thereof, will become a major factor in control of the world's birth rate. In a few countries initial steps have already been taken to accomplish this control.

2. The Pill itself, as well as its individual hormones, is used in the treatment and prevention of numerous menstrual problems that have troubled women for centuries. Prior to 1950, specific remedies were not available for the majority of ill-defined and little-understood "female disorders." Many, perhaps most, of these functional diseases seemed adequately treated with an earlier potion, Lydia Pinkham's tablets or tonic. Fortunately, the Pill provides more specific treatment and offers several advantages. In most women, the Pill produces a regular menstrual period with minimum bleeding. Therefore, it is highly effective in treating menstrual dysfunctions such as premenstrual tension, irregular or excessive bleeding, painful menstruation, and premenstrual breast tenderness.[1]

3. The Pill may be used to regulate the length of the menstrual cycle and thus permits the bleeding episode or "period" to occur at a planned and desirable time. It should be emphasized that the process of menstruation serves no useful function. Stated simply, menstruation occurs as the result of *not* becoming pregnant after ovulation. It does not, as believed in more superstitious days, rid the body of "poisons." Therefore, a significant number of women now choose not to menstruate at a specific time. Among them are swimmers, golfers, track stars, entertainers, and even women going on a vacation. The monthly "curse" or inconvenience may be delayed, safely, simply, and regularly.

4. The Pill might be considered a Godsend for the premeno-

pausal woman between the ages of forty-five and fifty-two. It prevents pregnancy at an age when most women have teenage daughters and sons. Some are grandmothers. Pregnancy is undesirable from several aspects. Medically, a patient in this age group has a markedly greater chance of developing complications during the pregnancy. The chances of birth defects such as mongolism are increased. Economically, a new pregnancy might necessitate the loss of a job for a working mother, or curtailment of educational funds for other members of the family.

The Pill has other advantages during the premenopausal years. Taken regularly, it prevents irregular bleeding and the occasional episodes of profuse bleeding that are due to the waning ovary's inability to ovulate normally. Since the bleeding that occurs after twenty days of the Pill is simply a "withdrawal" effect of the estrogen and progestin in the drug, the amount of flow is usually minimal. The lining of the womb just has not been stimulated to develop the thickness that occurs when ovulation occurs irregularly. Another bonus is provided since the womb lining cannot become overthickened or "hyperplastic," a condition which, if uncorrected, may eventually become cancerous.[2]

Many premenopausal women note symptoms of estrogen insufficiency as the ovary becomes a noncyclic organ in its secretion of hormones. The levels of estrogen in their bodies are described as "teetering," up one day, down the next. This is manifested by hot flashes, excessive perspiration, insomnia, and nervousness. If the estrogen remains low for several months, the lining of the vagina thins and small blood vessels disintegrate. This may cause spotting of blood after intercourse, and the lining becomes overly susceptible to infections. The net result is an inadequately lubricated, rather rigid vagina. Intercourse becomes painful and libido is reduced. The Pill provides excellent therapy for each of these symptoms.[3]

5. The Pill is used to improve infertility in women who have endometriosis or underdeveloped reproductive organs. In endometriosis, a disease of increasing incidence during the last fifty years, menstrual blood is ejected from the open ends of the tubes at the time of the normal period. This blood and fragments of

tissue from the womb lining (endometrium) are deposited on the ovaries and adjacent organs. Over a period of years, this misplaced tissue, called "endometriosis," is converted into scar tissue. The ovaries are unable to function normally and the tubes are incapable of picking up the egg at the time of ovulation. The best prevention and treatment of this disease is pregnancy. But many women, particularly during the early stages of the disease, are unmarried or are not desirous of pregnancy. If ovulation is suppressed for one or two years, the process of monthly spillage into the body cavity is interrupted and the areas of endometriosis are permitted to heal. The Pill produces this effect. In the treatment of this disease the estrogen-progestin pill is usually given *constantly* —not in the usual twenty-day cycles. The net result is called a "pseudopregnancy," since ovulation is suppressed, menstruation does not occur, and the levels of estrogen and progestin remain elevated—just as in normal pregnancy.[4] Dr. Allen Grant in Sydney, Australia, has used the cyclic, twenty-day method of pill administration for the treatment of endometriosis with excellent results.

Although long-term observations are not as yet available, I have suggested that the use of the Pill *for contraceptive purposes* in young women may actually *prevent* endometriosis. How? By diminishing the amount of blood ejected from the tubes each month. Many of the newer, more potent oral contraceptives result in very scanty periods. In some women the flow is entirely absent. Visualize this same process in the tubes. If the amount of material (blood and glands) oozing from the womb into the tubes is markedly reduced, the major factor causing the disease is prevented. During the last five years, I have been impressed by the low incidence of endometriosis in women who have used the Pill for three years or longer.

Some women are infertile because of inadequate hormonal stimulation, primarily estrogen and progesterone. Since these hormones stimulate growth of the womb and the tubes, prolonged deficiency causes these organs to be underdeveloped and incapable of maintaining pregnancy. Spontaneous abortion is common during the first 6 to 8 weeks. In some women, the endometrium is so thin that implantation of the fertilized egg is impossible. The

Pill, especially the sequential type, provides the needed estrogen to build the endometrium to a normal state and, during the last five days of the cycle, a progestin to produce a normal "withdrawal" flow. In many women classified as "habitual aborters" because they have had a minimum of three consecutive miscarriages during the first twelve weeks of pregnancy, use of the Pill for three to six months accomplishes two things.[5] First, it prevents pregnancy from occurring during the treatment period. Second, the hormones "prime" the endometrium to permit normal development and menstrual sloughing. Then, when pregnancy is planned, the uterus, endometrium and tubes are better prepared. As soon as pregnancy occurs, estrogens and progesterone are given to prevent miscarriage.

6. The Pill, both directly and indirectly, should be considered a major advance in preventing cancer in women. The chances of any woman developing cancer of the breast and female reproductive organs are about 10 per cent. Breast cancer occurs in about 5 per cent, and cancer of the vulva, vagina, cervix (neck of the womb), corpus (body of the womb), tubes, and ovaries account for the other 5 per cent.

The Pill has no direct effect, either beneficial or adverse, on the development of cancer of the breast or cervix, the two most common malignancies. That is to say, all of the statistical evidence available at the present time suggests no correlation between estrogen and the *cause* of breast cancer. There is, however, definite evidence that estrogen may *aggravate* breast cancer already present by stimulating its growth. No woman should take the Pill unless her breasts are regularly examined.

While the Pill has no direct effect on breast cancer, it has an indirect effect of great significance. The optimum therapy for breast cancer is early diagnosis. Surgery for early breast cancer produces a five-year survival rate of almost 90 per cent, whereas if the cancer has spread to adjacent lymph nodes, the five-year survival rate drops to 40 per cent. Surgery for late breast cancer is worthless, and all forms of treatment are merely palliative. It must be pointed out that the incidence and cure rate for breast cancer was exactly the same in 1965 as it was in 1930. Unless new

8   *Contraception*

treatment or diagnostic methods are developed, our only hope is early diagnosis. Considering the magnitude of the disease—one woman in every sixteen will eventually have breast cancer, making it the Number *1* cause of death in the age group forty-five to fifty-three; 25,000 deaths occur each year from breast cancer and 65,000 new cases are diagnosed each year—the physician has no greater responsibility than early diagnosis of this disease.

The Pill offers a great advantage in early diagnosis of breast cancer, for the user should appear twice a year (more often if indicated) at the doctor's office to have her prescription for pills refilled. At this time a routine examination permits the vital, early detection of breast cancer. The advantage the Pill offers in early detection of breast cancer is, I believe, a major step forward in preventive medicine, one that has not been widely publicized. I have detected minute masses in patients' breasts either at the time of their first visit, before any hormonal agent has been initiated, or at the time of the six-month checkup. Many of these were the size of a small pea; others were even smaller, but they were very early—and curable—cancer.

Cancer of the cervix is the second most common malignancy in women. One woman in every forty will develop this disease. Progress has been made, however, both in early diagnosis and in more effective treatment in the last thirty-five years. Yet almost 20,000 women die of this disease every year in the United States. This figure can and should be reduced, since many gynecologists are convinced that cancer of the cervix is a preventable disease.[6] How? By routine examinations and by the annual use of the Papanicolaou smear. The "Pap" smear detects abnormalities in cells shed from the cervix even before the disease occurs. Early treatment by cauterization, local removal, or hysterectomy prevents the development of cervical cancer. A woman taking the Pill and having an annual pelvic examination and Pap smear is almost completely protected from the disease. Furthermore, the hormones in the Pill do not affect already existing cervical cancer. Gynecologists have given estrogens to women who have been treated for this disease (by hysterectomy and removal of the ovaries or by x-ray and radium) for years. There is no evidence to suggest that estrogens affect the cure rate.

Cancer of the cervix occurs more commonly in women who have had sexual intercourse prior to the age of twenty, particularly if there have been multiple sexual partners. The disease is, therefore, rare in virgins but common in prostitutes. It also occurs more frequently in lower socio-economic groups, particularly the indigent. If a young girl, using the Pill, has frequent intercourse with multiple partners prior to age twenty, she has a statistically increased chance of getting cancer of the cervix. Since there is some evidence now that this cancer may be caused by a specific virus, possibly transmitted by the penis, the use of a diaphragm might offer some degree of protection. If the Pill is the sole reason for the increased frequency of intercourse, then it might be concluded that the Pill will cause an increased incidence of this disease. But the premalignant phase of cancer of the cervix, so called "cancer-in-situ" is easily detected by a routine "Pap" smear. Therefore, if a Pill user has a pelvic examination every six months and a "Pap" smear at least once a year, she can be certain that she will never develop "full-blown" cancer.

Suppose a study of Pill users in an indigent population group shows an increased number of patients with abnormal "Pap" smears and premalignant "cancer-in-situ." Does this mean that the Pill is related or causes these changes? Headlines might suggest that this is so. But it is necessary to show an increased *incidence* in the Pill users over the natural high-*prevalence* rate in this group before this conclusion is warranted. Screening of the non-Pill users of the same age, same number of children, same sexual habits, and same racial background must be done simultaneously and in a prospective fashion. Conclusions cannot be based on a comparison of Pill users *now* with the *previous* incidence of non-Pill users.

If the Pill has a marked *indirect* advantage in permitting early diagnosis of the two most common forms of cancer in women, it has a *direct* advantage in preventing cancer of the endometrium, the third most common malignancy. There will be further discussion of this in Chapter 14, but at this preliminary point it may be said that the accepted therapy, worldwide, for widespread endometrial cancer is the administration of a synthetic progestin. The agents used are Depo-Provera and Delalutin, two particularly potent progestins with properties very similar to those of the ovarian hormone progesterone. In 1959, the remarkable effect of these progestins upon premalignant phases of endometrial cancer were reported.[2] Even if the cancer had spread to the lungs, abdomen, and pelvis, the progestin therapy was effective in producing a remission of the disease in one-third of the patients. Some patients so treated are still alive! Progestin therapy for endometrial malignancy is an important breakthrough in the field of gynecological cancer.*[7]

It seems logical to me that if progestin is used to treat existing endometrial cancer, then it should be useful in *preventing* its development. While none of the brands of the Pill now marketed contains Depo-Provera or Delalutin, all the brands contain a progestin that is similar, if less potent. One of the effects of a progestin is that it is anti-estrogenic—and some physicians believe that cancer of the endometrium may be related, in part, to prolonged estrogen stimulation. This hormone, some believe, causes an overthickening or hyperplasia of the endometrium that may lead to cancer. The progestin in the Pill prevents this hyperplasia from developing.[8] Therefore, those women who might develop cancer of the womb lining from hyperplasia will be protected— since the hyperplasia does not occur.

7. The Pill, because it is so effective, has diminished the number of therapeutic abortions. In the past, the majority of these were performed at the recommendation of a psychiatrist and obstetrician, both of whom agreed that continuation of the pregnancy would have a deleterious effect on the health of the mother. Now, effective planning by the patient and her consultants can prevent these pregnancies. Hopefully, the number of criminal abortions will also be reduced. In certain locales progress in this direction

---

* A less well-known use for Depo-Provera and Delalutin is the prevention of pregnancy in the rape victim. The progestin is injected directly on the lining of the uterus. Within minutes, the endometrium is changed so markedly that implantation of the fertilized egg is impossible. Time favors the use of this method since the fertilized egg needs three days to traverse the tube; then it "free floats" in the uterus for three more days before implanting in the womb. It is not a treatment to be used indiscriminately or with any frequency, but it is a method of preventing the ultimate tragedy that befalls a rape victim.

has also been made. For example, in a large metropolitan city in South America, the number of criminal abortions performed each year exceeded the number of live births. Even worse, the number of women who died from infections caused by criminal abortions was almost 50 percent. In 1963, I visited this city with two other physicians who had extensive experience with the Pill and family planning. After a series of lectures to local physicians, a planned-parenthood clinic was established and the Pill was distributed to those desirous of participating in the program. Within a year the number of criminal abortions and maternal deaths had dropped precipitously, and a continued downward trend is evident.

8. Another major advantage of the Pill has been its effect on the number of women undergoing a hysterectomy for benign diseases. I have already mentioned endometriosis as an example of a disease that may be managed by the use of hormones and whose very development may actually be prevented by prolonged use of the Pill.[1, 3] Irregular and profuse bleeding during the premenopause has been a major cause of hysterectomy in the past. If this bleeding is due to abnormal ovarian function, surgery may be avoided by placing the ovary at rest and substituting the hormones of the Pill for malfunction of ovarian hormones. While no reports are available to tell us the number of patients who have avoided hysterectomy by proper hormonal treatment, I would estimate the total to be in the thousands. Perhaps even tens of thousands.

9. The final advantages of the Pill may be grouped under a very inclusive term, "psychological factors." Many women have described their marriages and themselves as happier while taking the oral contraceptive. Women with hormone imbalance or menstrual disturbance say "they just feel better." Others have noted greater enjoyment of intercourse, both because of increased libido and absence of the fear of pregnancy. If you are one of the many thousands of women who have noted this improved feeling, a new zest for living, a *joie de vivre,* you might ask why, or how does it happen? The reason is simple. Painful menstruation, the associated backache, leg ache, sore breasts, and the myriad symptoms grouped under the term "premenstrual tension" are all due to the process of ovulation and the subsequent secretion of the

hormone progesterone from the ovary. Women who do not ovulate do not have these complaints. For many years before the Pill was even thought of, I treated these complaints by suppression of ovulation with estrogen tablets—and the results were excellent.[9] Consider, then, the advantages of the Pill to the woman who has the unholy triad of painful periods that are frequently profuse, premenstrual tension, and a fear of pregnancy bordering on schizophrenia. Not only is she protected from pregnancy, she has the knowledge that her periods will occur regularly (or at a specific time if she so desires); she need not fear the embarrassment of profuse bleeding and flooding; and she is spared the discomfort and the associated tensions that have for too long been considered a necessary part of her femininity.

In spite of this imposing list of advantages of the Pill, there is still consistent criticism leveled against it. This criticism has been of several types. First, exaggerated magazine scare stories and exposés have frequently served to confuse and frighten the reader. Some magazines have furnished the reader with excellent and forthright reviews, giving both pro and con arguments. Unfortunately, not enough of these have appeared to balance the damage done by the early, less accurate articles. Run-of-the-mill news items concerning the Pill are almost always front-page material, but they are necessarily brief. More important medical news is usually relegated to an unobtrusive spot, if printed at all.

A second type of criticism comes from qualified physicians and researchers. A survey of 6,733 physicians conducted in 1967 by the American College of Obstetricians and Gynecologists showed that fifty-eight physicians of those questioned never prescribe the Pill. A total of 5.2 per cent said they prescribe it only for noncontraceptive purposes, that is, for control of menstrual and other female disorders. A total of 92.1 percent said they prescribe the Pill for both contraceptive and noncontraceptive purposes. Among those surveyed, 87.3 per cent said they prescribe oral contraceptives more frequently than any other type of contraceptive. Thus, the number of physicians *not* prescribing the Pill is small and, as the survey showed, the overwhelming majority of nonprescribers did so primarily for religious reasons. Only 1 per cent of physicians said they did not use the Pill in their practice because of concern about its safety. This is indeed a rarity—to get 99 per cent of physicians to agree on any medical problem.

Small in number though they may be, it is entirely appropriate and desirable that physicians express their concern about the safety of the Pill. Most of these doctors are uneasy about the long-term effects of the medication. There are certain questions about long-term effects that can now be answered if "long term" is defined as ten years. Some patients have actually been taking the Pill for twelve years without apparent ill effects. Yet, there are some investigators and clinicians who state that "The Pill cannot be considered safe until it has been used for 20, 30 or even 40 years. It takes that long for certain forms of cancer to develop." My reaction to this objection is simple. I doubt very much whether any woman will take the Pill, as we now know it, for twenty or thirty years. Newer agents, injectable substances, vaccines, and a host of potent compounds, will undoubtedly replace the Pill during the next decade. Furthermore, if the Pill takes forty years to produce a cancer in the human female, it is indeed a weak agent. Much less potent than the cigarette!

A third type of criticism of the Pill, and probably the most devastating in regard to the confidence of the patient, is misinterpretation, by newspaper or magazine writers, of specific facts presented by physicians in medical articles. While it is possible that these writers have presented alarming and confused data to the reader because of their own ignorance of the subject, it is also possible that conclusions have been reported out of context to gain front-page acceptance. For example, it was reported on the front page of every major newspaper in the United States in 1965 that a number of women taking oral contraceptives were found to have certain eye defects. The possibility of blindness was mentioned. This was of grave concern to patients taking the Pill and to the gynecologists who prescribe them. Many women immediately discontinued the Pill and undoubtedly a good many became pregnant. But the unanswered question was whether or not the reported eye defects were caused by the medication or were just coincidental findings.

A study was organized immediately by Dr. Elizabeth Connell

at the New York Medical College.[10] Her surprising findings were that 580 (73.4 per cent) of 790 women had eye abnormalities *before* starting the Pill. Dr. Connell subsequently reported in the medical literature that "The number of abnormalities we found in our control patients was entirely unanticipated. The majority were not pathological in the sense that they produced visual damage. However, their presence in a retrospective study could readily lead to erroneous conclusions about eye damage related to the use of oral contraceptives." She suggested that more study and observation was needed and cautioned, "It would appear important not to overestimate the amount of damage caused by the Pill in light of the findings in so-called normal patients." The question is whether women who read the original news item linking eye defects to the Pill also read Dr. Connell's report. Probably not, since it was published primarily in medical newspapers and magazines.

Another example: In 1967, a team of physicians at Western Reserve University in Cleveland, Ohio, reported that a group of women with a previous history of migraine headaches had developed strokes after taking the Pill. Their reports made headlines. What tended to be lost in the reports was the fact that strokes were reported in only nine patients. These were patients referred to a specialty clinic from many areas. Unless the total number of patients taking the Pill in those areas is reported along with the number who developed stroke, a statistical correlation cannot be determined. In other words, how many patients developed stroke who were *not* taking the Pill? The researchers did not state that there was a causal relationship between the Pill and strokes. They were cognizant of the fact that numerous other factors might have caused this serious illness. Whereas the physicians merely recorded an observation, the newspaper versions implied a correlation to the reader.

A more recent and glaring example of the application of journalistic "scare" techniques to the Pill involves press reports of a British study "linking" increased incidence of thromboembolism (blood clots) to use of the Pill.[11, 12] Briefly recapitulated, the British statistical study showed that a user of the Pill has a sixfold greater chance of death from thromboembolism than the non-user. This "fact" was seized by the popular press and prominently displayed. Many press stories did not report, as the British study did, that the incidence was still extremely small and that a British woman's chance of death during pregnancy was seventeen times greater than if she took the Pill. Nor did the journalists follow up their original stories to report the widespread criticism of the statistical techniques used in the British study or to give equal space to subsequent studies that showed fatalities from thromboembolism to be lower among Pill users than nonusers.[13]

Because the Pill is being taken by over 6 million women in the United States alone, it is inevitable that any disease, discomfort, or unusual symptom that occurs will be linked to the contraceptive. Users of the Pill are just as susceptible to disease, accidents, or injuries as nonusers. It is logical to assume, therefore, that every disease, injury, or surgical emergency will occur in users in the same frequency as in nonusers. If leg cramps develop in a woman taking the Pill, her first thought is that she has a blood clot that might spread to the lungs and kill her. But if the same leg cramp develops in a woman *not* taking the Pill, she is likely to ascribe her symptoms to a new pair of high heel shoes or a game of tennis or just plain overwork. The former patient will rush to her physician; the latter rarely does. If both have thrombophlebitis, a localized blood clot in the veins of the leg, it is obvious that the incidence of admissions to hospitals will be higher in women who are taking the Pill.

When the various ailments apparently due to the use of the Pill are combined, the nonmedical reader is confused beyond her ability to interpret fact from fantasy. Blood clots, blindness, migraine headaches, strokes, jaundice, cancer! The end of such illogical reasoning was illustrated in the recent ACOG** survey. Gynecologists reported that a frequent cause for discontinuing the Pill was fear and fear alone. I must comment that this has not been so in my practice. Perhaps I have been able to dispel fear. Fear is dependent upon ignorance. Children fear the unusual, the dark, the unexplored. But ignorance is dissipated by knowledge,

** American College of Obstetricians and Gynecologists.

by experience, by exploration. My patients do not fear the diseases so widely advertised in the press. Why should they? No one has as yet shown them reason to do so. A recent issue of *McCall's* magazine describes why 3 million women quit taking the Pill. The article is based on a study by Professor Charles F. Westoff of Princeton University and Professor Norman B. Ryder of the University of Wisconsin. According to this report, about 20 per cent of the women stopped the Pill because they desired to become pregnant, were divorced or separated, entered the menopause, or were estranged from their husbands because of war or business. Of the remaining 80 percent, 15 per cent listed psychological factors— worry, fear, distrust of the efficacy of the medication; 65 per cent indicated that unpleasant side effects were the major reason for discontinuing the Pill. But several points of importance were clarified in this report. First of all, more women under the age of thirty continued the Pill and, rather strangely, twice as many older women gave it up than did their younger sisters. As might be expected, most of the drop-outs occurred during the first three months of pill taking—when the incidence of side effects is the highest. The incidence of drop-outs was higher among less-educated women, actually being twice as high in women who had not completed high school. There is no racial pattern among drop-outs, and Westoff and Ryder found practically no difference between the rate of drop-outs between non-whites and whites.

DISADVANTAGES

1. Medication is being given to a healthy woman. It is the essence of good medical practice to prescribe medication only when necessary and then to administer as little of it as possible to secure the desired effect. A physician strives to give drugs only if a specific need is present.

2. Side effects do occur. Each of these will be subsequently discussed, but at this point it may be said that since the Pill contains the hormones of pregnancy, estrogen and progestin, users tend to react in a manner similar to a natural pregnancy. Some women feel wonderful. Others experience weight gain, nausea, sore breasts, and depression. These side effects usually disappear

within a month or two as the body adjusts to the higher hormone levels. Some effects of the hormones may be more long lasting, particularly darkening of the skin. These changes of skin pigmentation occur during pregnancy and are known as the "mask of pregnancy." There may be an increased tendency toward varicose veins among users. It must be emphasized, however, that the serious and occasionally fatal complications of pregnancy, such as infection, toxemia, and hemorrhage are not associated with use of the Pill.

3. The Pill prevents ovulation. Since this is the primary purpose of the Pill, it may seem strange to list it as a disadvantage. Suppressing ovulation on a short-term basis is no problem. There is abundant evidence that short-term users who go off the Pill ovulate normally and become pregnant without delay. The concern is with the long-term user—and I must emphasize the word *concern*. The concern is that after a prolonged period of suppressed ovulation a woman might not be able to ovulate again. The evidence to date indicates the concern is overrated. A very few women have noted irregular ovulation or lack of ovulation after discontinuing the Pill. Although the exact incidence is not known, I doubt that it is higher than the same problem occurring after pregnancy. Most of these had irregular periods before using oral contraceptives. In my experience ovulation usually recurs in about six to eight months. If it does not, a new drug, clomiphene, is capable of restarting the ovulatory process. Observations of women who have had ovarian tumors that secreted large amounts of estrogen indicate the reversibility of the process. After surgical removal of the tumors, ovulation begins again and pregnancies occur without difficulty. Even so, it must be said that an ideal oral contraceptive would be one that did not suppress ovulation.

4. There are psychological and moral disadvantages. Some women have reported a loss of sexual desire while taking the Pill, which created a strain on their marriage and affected their sense of well-being. Some observers feel the Pill encourages promiscuity. While I don't share this view, it is a possible disadvantage.

Some readers may be surprised that I have not listed "dangers" of cancer and pulmonary embolism among the disadvantages. I believe one of the advantages of the Pill is that it prevents uterine cancer and permits early detection of cancer of the breast and cervix. There is some evidence of increased incidence of blood-clotting disorders among Pill users, but the risks for a woman who becomes pregnant are considerably greater. *Deaths* from blood clots spreading to the lungs occur in 1.5 per 100,000 pill users age 20–34 and in 3.9 per 100,000 pill users age 35–44. In nonusers the incidence is 0.2 and 0.5 per 100,000. But deaths during pregnancy, from all causes, are 22.8 per 100,000 in the age groups 20–34 and 57.6 per 100,000 between ages 35–44. The risk of death is higher from driving a car, crossing the street, or smoking cigarettes excessively. Since the Pill is *the* most effective contraceptive available today, it is difficult to see how any slight tendency toward thrombophlebitis or blood clots in the lung (pulmonary emboli) can be listed as a disadvantage.

CONCLUSIONS

It seems to me that the advantages of the Pill far outweigh the disadvantages. This comparison of risk undoubtedly accounts for the fact that the overwhelming majority of obstetricians and gynecologists prescribe it.

Returning to the question of whether the fears of the Pill are justified, it must be emphasized that oral contraceptives are perhaps the most thoroughly tested medication ever marketed in this country. Hundreds of thousands of animal experiments have been performed. The most thorough study of Pill users has been in progress in Puerto Rico since 1956. Millions of users are closely observed by their physicians. The Federal Food and Drug Administration has imposed the most careful scrutiny on the Pill and its various manufacturers since its inception. In 1966, the FDA impaneled an Advisory Committee under the chairmanship of Dr. Louis M. Hellman, Professor of Obstetrics and Gynecology at the State University of New York. This committee studied the drugs, their manufacture and effects, and concluded: "The Committee finds no adequate scientific data, at this time, proving these compounds unsafe for human use."

Nonetheless, fear of the Pill persists. In a way this is good, since fear has prevented complacency. It has spurred exhaustive research, so that we know today not only that the oral contraceptives work but also rather precisely *how* they work. This contrasts with a drug such as aspirin. Despite its decades of use, no one quite knows how aspirin relieves pain, reduces fever, or alleviates arthritis. The fear has also been a spur to research on improved methods of contraception. Great progress has been made, and the next decade will witness a multifaceted approach to the problem of conception control.

Yet, in another way, the vague, widespread fear of the Pill is difficult to understand. Its side effects are far less frequent and severe than those associated with such medications as penicillin, cortisone, or aspirin, with which little public fear is associated. This country has a greater health problem from overuse of vitamins and cigarettes than it has from oral contraceptives. Allergic reactions to deodorant soaps have been described as epidemic in the United States, yet no great fear of cleanliness has resulted. Fear of the Pill persists despite the fact that it produces few allergic reactions. It is difficult to equate the fear of cancer associated with the Pill in the light of conclusive data linking cancer with cigarette smoking.

Psychology and psychiatry are not my specialties, but I feel that perhaps the fear of oral contraceptives is rooted in some form of guilt about using them. Perhaps bearing children and reproducing the species is such a basic function of man that deliberately preventing it results in guilt. Or, perhaps the ancient precept of the Judeo-Christian religions that sex is intended for reproduction and not for pleasure lingers enough to create guilt.

Having children has always been considered a virtue, although, with the population crisis, childbearing is becoming less and less virtuous. Yet the fact remains that man, throughout his history, has tried almost as hard *not* to have children as he has to have them. The fascinating story of contraception through the ages begins the next chapter.

2. Methods of Contraception

THE WIVES OF North African desert tribesmen mixed gunpowder solution and foam from a camel's mouth and drank the potion. Egyptian women inserted pessaries made from crocodile dung into the vagina or used tampons made from lint soaked in fermented acacia juice. The Chinese fried quicksilver in oil and drank it, or swallowed fourteen live tadpoles three days after menstruation. Greek women of the second century made vaginal plugs of wool soaked in sour oil, honey, cedar gum, pomegranate, and fig pulp. Others ate the uterus of a female mule. Byzantine women of the sixth century attached a tube containing cat liver to their left foot. In the Middle Ages, potions were prepared from willow leaves, iron rust or slag, clay, and the kidney of a mule. European brides of the seventeenth century were instructed to sit on their fingers while riding in their coaches or to place roasted walnuts in the bosom, one for every barren year desired.

These are but a few of the more picturesque methods of "contraception" used in man's efforts to achieve family planning.[14] Obviously, the unwanted child was of as much concern to the ancients as to modern man. More successful, and more sanitary, methods of conception control are now available, based on our knowledge of how conception and pregnancy occur.

The process of conception is so precise that it is amazing it happens so often. Stated simply, conception occurs when an ovum, or egg, is fertilized by a male spermatozoan, or sperm. But the process is infinitely more complicated. The sperm are suspended in a liquid called seminal fluid. This fluid is ejaculated into the vagina, where it reaches a small opening in the lowermost portion of the uterus, the cervix. The number of sperm ejaculated varies, but in a normal individual there are hundreds of millions in each cubic centimeter of fluid. The total amount of fluid ejaculated is about four cubic centimeters or one teaspoonful, so the total number of sperm may reach 1 billion. At the time of ovulation the cervix contains a clear, watery mucus that is an excellent habitat for the sperm, permitting their survival for as long as a week.

The sperm swim up the cervical canal—no one knows why they do not swim down—a distance of about one inch and enter the uterus. The uterus, or womb, is about the size of a small pear in a woman who has never had children and about the size of a medium sized pear in those who have. The sperm swim rapidly up the cavity of the uterus and into the Fallopian tubes. Considering their microscopic size, the sperm move with great rapidity and within an hour reach the outer portion of the tubes, which are in close proximity to the ovaries. At the time of ovulation the open ends of the tubes are actually grasping the ovary awaiting the expulsion of the egg. This is one reason that a douche is a completely unsatisfactory method of contraception. Chances are the sperm are already in the uterus by the time the douche is taken and cannot be washed out. In any event, sperm that reach the open end of the tubes may live for days awaiting the appearance of the egg.

A woman having a regular twenty-eight-day menstrual cycle normally ovulates on or about the fourteenth day of the cycle. The first day of menstruation is called Day 1 of the menstrual cycle. For some unknown reason, women always tabulate from the day the menstrual period ends. Try to think about it this way. It may take anywhere from seven to twenty-one days to permit the follicle growing in the ovary to mature. But once ovulation occurs, menstruation will occur in fourteen to sixteen days. The later phase of the cycle, the "postovulatory phase," is constant; the preovulatory phase is frequently irregular, and may last sixty to ninety days. Furthermore, although the "average" menstrual cycle is supposed to last twenty-eight days, the majority of women do not have a maintained, clock-like rhythm. Cycles of twenty-one to thirty-five days are perfectly normal and occur frequently. Furthermore, any number of factors such as stress, worry, geographic changes, and tranquilizing drugs can produce shortening or lengthening of the cycle. Even excessive weight gain or loss may do the same thing. I have seen numerous examples of women whose husbands were suddenly called to military service who either stopped ovulating and menstruating entirely or whose day of ovulation was delayed. If a woman whose usual cycle was twenty-eight days did not ovulate until Day 21 of the cycle, the period would occur 14 days later, making a cycle of thirty-five days.

At the time the egg is released from the follicle, several things happen. A muscular ligament between the uterus and the ovary contracts in such a way as to move the ovary slightly behind and under the uterus. It is then in a closer position to the tube. Then, the finger-like projections at the end of the tubes, called fimbria, undulate and sweep across the ovary and grasp it—the so-called "tubal embrace." When the egg is released from the ovary, it floats out in a stream of fluid from its own ruptured follicle. The tubal fingers engulf the egg much like the tentacles of an octopus grasping its prey. The egg remains in this area only momentarily since the tiny hairs, or cilia, propel the egg into the tubal opening, and it is sucked into the tubal canal. If intercourse has been timed properly, myriads of sperm surround and attack the capsule that surrounds the egg. Why only one sperm is capable of penetrating the capsule and all others are repelled remains one of the major mysteries of conception.

If fertilization has occurred on Day 14, the fertilized egg, or zygote, spends the next three days descending the tube and the next three days (18, 19, and 20) floating freely in the cavity of the uterus. During this time, several things are happening. The zygote is growing. One, then two, then dozens, then hundreds of cell divisions occur. Important hormonal changes are taking place that will prepare an optimum spot in the uterus so that the egg may implant. Estrogen and progesterone from the ruptured follicle, now called the corpus luteum, or yellow body, stimulate the lining of the uterus so that it becomes much thicker. The blood supply is increased and glands grow, branch, and prepare the pablum for the parasitic zygote, which will forage voraciously for nutriment soon after it imbeds.

By the seventh day after fertilization, the endometrium is ready to receive and nourish the zygote, which is now just barely visible to the naked eye. When the zygote is securely attached to the endometrium, implantation is said to have occurred. Precision is necessary for effective implantation. Timing is all important. Although it is not known why the fertilized egg floats in the cavity of the uterus for three days, it is probably related to the condition of the endometrium. For example, if the endometrium matures too quickly, the zygote cannot burrow into the "overripe" tissue. It is expelled with the menstrual flow. Conversely, if the endometrium lags in its development, due to inadequate estrogen and progesterone, the egg will find the soil barren and fail to implant. Thus, the major cause of early miscarriages is failure of implantation. These "spontaneous abortions" are never known to the individual but may account for a temporary period of infertility in many newly married couples. The second most common factor is that of improper or inadequate implantation, resulting in loss of the zygote through menstruation. Frequently, in women having this problem, the menstrual period may be delayed for seven to ten days. When it does occur, the flow is excessive and may be accompanied by more crampy pain than usual. If a curettage of the uterus is done at this time, the gynecologist is able to make the correct diagnosis by microscopic examination of the tissue.

As the normal process of ovulation and implantation is known, it is now relatively simple to devise methods for effective contraception.

CONDOMS

During the sixteenth century, the Italian anatomist Fallopius, for whom the Fallopian tubes are named, devised a linen sheath for the penis, an effective forerunner to the condom. Although Fallopius advised use of the condom to prevent the spread of syphilis, it was not widely accepted. Madame de Sevigné, in a letter to her daughter in 1671, called the condom an "armor against enjoyment and a spider web against danger." Casanova, in his *Memoires,* indicates he used condoms both to prevent venereal disease and to avoid impregnating his women. He was not a fan, however. "I do not care to shut myself up in a piece of dead skin in order to prove I am perfectly alive." Although used extensively in the brothels of the eighteenth century, the condom could not be manufactured in quantity until vulcanization of rubber was developed about the middle of the nineteenth century. Today, about 700 to 800 million are produced annually in the United States.[15]

The condom, as used today, is a covering for the penis, usually made of thin rubber and sometimes previously lubricated. It is designed to capture and hold the seminal fluid, thus preventing its deposition in the vagina and over the cervix. The condom has the added advantage of preventing venereal disease.

There are several objections to the condom. First, it must be applied prior to intercourse. If this application occurs between sexual foreplay and coitus, this frequently annoys both partners. The annoying interlude may cause diminution in erection, particularly in men with borderline impotence. In older males, it frequently diminishes sensation so as to make ejaculation difficult and even impossible. The woman may complain of dulled sensation or inability to sense the ejaculatory process. The biggest difficulty with the condom as a contraceptive is that the thin sheath may rupture or loosen, allowing sperm to enter the vagina. Also, pregnancies have resulted from premature ejaculation by the male prior to use of the condom.

COITUS INTERRUPTUS

This is the oldest of the useful methods of contraception. The male withdraws his penis prior to ejaculation. There are several problems, however. Although the numbers of sperm in the fluid ejaculated may total 1 billion, only one is necessary for fertilization. A few sperm are usually present in the lubricating fluids secreted from the penis during sexual excitement. It is possible that several sperm may be on their way to the uterus well before ejaculation. Moreover, a great deal of coital experience and willpower must be employed by the male to enforce this method. The penis must be completely withdrawn, not only from the vagina but from the external genitalia as well. It is a little-known fact that pregnancy may occur from ejaculation into or on the labia and, since the female may gain satisfaction from the male's ejaculation against the clitoris, this practice is common. Withdrawal does not, unfortunately, guarantee avoidance of pregnancy.

RHYTHM METHOD

The basic principle of rhythm is the avoidance of coitus during the time when the woman is ovulating. As a practical method of contraception, however, several difficulties are encountered. There is no way at present, despite extensive research, to determine with precision when ovulation occurs. One index frequently used is to chart the basal body temperature. A slight dip in temperature is frequently seen at the time of ovulation, and this is followed by a maintained rise after it. The temperature rise is due to the progesterone secreted by the corpus luteum after ovulation. Progesterone is thermogenic, even when given to males, and the maintenance of the temperature rise, followed by a fall just prior to menstruation, is a fairly good index of ovulation. It is not proof, however. Only pregnancy is proof of ovulation.

Even though a woman ovulates regularly on the fourteenth day of a twenty-eight-day cycle, a considerable margin of time must be allowed for safety. Under the most ideal circumstances, intercourse should be avoided from the eleventh day to the eighteenth day of each cycle. But even a week's abstinence is no insurance, for sperm may survive for several days, perhaps even longer inside the female genital tract. Pregnancies have occurred after a single coitus seven days prior to apparent ovulation as indicated by the basal body temperature. If ovulation is early or late, the risks of pregnancy are greatly compounded.

A simple formula may be used to calculate the fertile period. A woman should record her menstrual cycles for at least one year. The number 18 is subtracted from the number of days in the shortest cycle and 11 is subtracted from the longest cycle. The days in between are considered fertile or unsafe. For example, if the cycle varies between 25 and 32 days, 25 minus 18 equal 7, and 32 minus 11 equal 21. This means a two-week period of abstinence each month, a degree of deprivation unacceptable to most newly married couples whose average frequency of coitus is three to four times weekly. Because of the long life of some sperm, there is still a small risk of pregnancy even if abstinence is observed from the seventh to the twenty-first day of the cycle.

VAGINAL SPERMICIDES

These are preparations, marketed as foams, creams, or synthetic gels, that are inserted in the vagina against the cervix with a plastic applicator. They act by destroying sperm without harming the delicate vaginal lining. Only one application is required before each night of intercourse, but the jelly or foam must be in place at least three minutes. Their effectiveness is minimal after one hour.

VAGINAL DIAPHRAGMS WITH SPERMICIDES

The diaphragm was developed over forty years ago by a European physician and consists of a circular metal spring covered with fine latex rubber. The spring is flexible along one axis and the entire diaphragm can be compressed and easily passed into the vagina. It is then released in the upper and larger portion of the vagina, where it covers the cervix completely. Since the dimensions of the vagina from the area behind the cervix to the pubic bone vary, diaphragms are available in specific sizes. This distance may be measured by vaginal examination, and the proper size prescribed. To increase the effectiveness of the diaphragm, it should be covered with a spermicidal jelly or cream. When the diaphragm is inserted properly, it will completely cover the cervix and cause no discomfort. A properly fitted diaphragm will be unnoticed by the male partner. It should be inserted prior to intercourse and, preferably, be removed six to eight hours later, usually the next morning.

A woman using a diaphragm has a 10 to 12 per cent chance of becoming pregnant during the space of one year. Improper insertion, imperfect materials, and forgetfulness probably account for most pregnancies.

INTRAUTERINE DEVICES

The methods described thus far prevent the sperm from reaching the egg. Intrauterine devices (IUD) utilize a different principle, and although the precise mechanism of action is still unknown, over six million women throughout the world have used these devices during the last five years. IUD's are made of soft, flexible plastic molded into various sizes and shapes. They are inserted by a physician into the uterus, where they may remain for indefinite periods. Although the original devices were much less effective in conception control than the Pill, newer ones are now available that may afford almost complete protection. In one recent study, a double-coil device was found to be comparable to oral contraceptives. In patients with low motivation for pill taking, such as the indigent population in the United States or in India or China, the double coil may prove to be the method of choice. Another new stainless steel IUD, which looks like a bunch of paper clips strung together, has demonstrated a substantial improvement in effectiveness. Spontaneous expulsions were noted in only 1 per cent of patients, and the need to remove the device occurred in only 5 per cent.

The intrauterine device is not new. It was used in Germany at least forty years ago, but the method was discontinued because infection of the uterus and tubes often resulted. But these early devices were made of metal. Today's plastic devices have alleviated many of the problems. Three major types are available. The Spiral is equipped with a small beadlike protuberance that extends out of the cervix into the vagina. The Loop is equipped with two small threads that extend into the vagina for identification. The Bow is so called because it resembles a bow tie.

Experience thus far indicates that the Loop and a newer product, the Saf-T-Coil, are superior to the other devices. In comparison to the Loop, the pregnancy and perforation (of the uterus) rates are high with the Bow, expulsions and side effects are common with the Coil, and the pregnancy rate is high and insertion and removal difficult with the steel ring. An advantage of the Saf-T-Coil is that it is available in a presterilized package.

The pregnancy rate declines with time. It is about 2.4 per cent during the first year, 2 per cent during the second year, and 1 per cent thereafter. Two out of three pregnancies occur with the device still in the uterus, and one-third are associated with unnoticed expulsion. Pregnancies with the device in place are associated with an abortion rate of about 33 per cent. Pregnancies that go to term are not associated with a higher-than-normal rate of fetal deformity.

The expulsion rate of the Loop is about 10 per cent during the first year, falling to 2.5 per cent in the second year, 1.5 per cent in the third, and less than 1 per cent thereafter. Generally speaking, the shorter the interval between delivery and IUD insertion, the higher the rate of expulsion. The ideal time for insertion of the IUD is when the patient returns for her six-week check-up, since then her motivation is high and the procedure is relatively easy. Ideally, the IUD wearer should be examined after the first menstrual period following insertion in order to detect early expulsion; after the third menstrual period in order to deal with early side effects; and at annual intervals thereafter. The wearer should examine herself at weekly intervals, and especially after each menstrual period.

Considerable research has been performed in an effort to determine how the intrauterine devices work. One explanation suggests that the IUD prevents pregnancy by speeding the fertilized egg through the tube. Thus, it arrives in the uterus before the endometrium is prepared for implantation. If this is the correct mechanism of action, the IUD's may be classified as an abortifacient. An abortifacient, that is, of a fertilized but unimplanted egg. Since definitions of the beginning of life have varied throughout the centuries, even in the Roman Catholic Church, it is probably more correct to describe the mechanism as "implantation prevention." A more recent theory, based on animal investigation, suggests that the lining of the uterus produces a toxin, or poison, that either kills sperm on their way up, or kills fertilized eggs on their way down.

The IUD is useful in certain women who find mechanical methods too messy and too demanding. These women are not adequately motivated to use a diaphragm or cream. Others have persistent Pill side effects. Intrauterine devices are less effective than the Pill, and they may produce disturbing symptoms, such as abnormal bleeding and pain. Furthermore, serious complications have occurred. Rupture of the uterus and pelvic infection have occasionally necessitated hysterectomy in young women. These are rare complications and probably were caused by improper technique when inserted.

The intrauterine device should not be used in the presence of uterine fibroids, or if irregular or unexplained bleeding has been noted. Congenital abnormalities of the uterus and infection of the cervix or vagina also are contraindications to their insertion. In some instances, the IUD has been placed in a uterus containing an unknown (or known) pregnancy. Abortion usually results and may be followed by infection, peritonitis, and sterility. The IUD's are difficult to insert in women who have not had children, usually because the cervical opening is so small. However, once the device has remained in place for twenty-four hours, performance in terms of pregnancy rates, expulsions, and removals for reason of comfort proves about the same for women who have borne children and women who have not. This has been the experience of Dr. Christopher Tietze, Associate Director of the Biomedical Division of the Population Council.[17]

A major disadvantage of the IUD is the high rate of "fall out," which may go unnoticed. Therefore the patient must examine her-

self vaginally once weekly to be certain the device is still in place.*
Many women complain of menstrual cramps during the first two
or three periods after insertion. The cramps may increase in severity, necessitating removal of the device. Excessive and irregular
bleeding, if recurrent, also demand removal.

The Advisory Committee on Obstetrics and Gynecology to The
Federal Food and Drug Administration has recently concluded
a year-long study of intrauterine devices. They found "adequate
scientific data attesting to their effectiveness and utility" but
warned that their insertion "carries a definite, albeit small, risk of
infection and uterine perforation." This committee evaluated the
data from 27,600 women covering more than 477,000 woman-
months of insertion. They found the IUD's to be "far more reliable"
than the diaphragm and condom and "only slightly less reliable
than the oral compounds." They noted that the expulsion rate declined steeply with age, and less steeply with the number of previous pregnancies. Thus a woman in her thirties having had only
one previous child would have less chance of expelling the device
than a woman in her twenties who had had five children. The
expulsion rate varied inversely with the size of the device and was
higher during the first few months after insertion. The committee
indicated a mortality of 0.2 per 10,000 insertions, due usually to
perforation of the uterus (the mortality rate due to lung clots in
pill users has been given as 0.13 per 10,000 [ages 18–34] and 0.34
per 10,000 [ages 35–44]).

In summary, the IUD has not approached original expectations,
but improvements in design are certain to provide better acceptance. At the moment the greatest market for IUD's is in underdeveloped countries. Since the devices are cheap and may be
utilized for years, crash programs were instituted almost five years
ago. But health officials in certain countries are not exactly enthusiastic about them. Dr. L. S. Sodhy[18] of Kuala Lumpur, Malaysia, has commented,

---

* Gynecologists at Johns Hopkins Hospital in Baltimore devised a magnetized
IUD and furnished the patient with a small compass. When the compass was
placed over the pubic area, the needle rotated and indicated that the device
was in place. It has been suggested that a vigorous compass swing to the north
indicated a "yes," whereas a feeble variation to the south meant a definite "no."

The IUD at first appeared to possess qualities superior to those of the oral contraceptive. Its application seemed so simple that it was hoped and believed that we had got nearer to the ideal contraceptive. When, however, it was introduced into some of the clinics of the [Malaysian] Federation, its disadvantages began to show. It requires doctors and nurses for fitting, and after fitting to cope with many complaints. Although it is inexpensive, the cost of insertion and after care is high, especially in Malaysia where medical personnel is in short supply.

. . . Trials on the IUD started about two years ago. Since then a few IUD clinics have been started, but at present the response is not encouraging and it will be some time before an assessment can be made. To conclude, I would state that in Malaysia the oral contraceptive is now the main method of family planning, and has been largely responsible for more people adopting family planning.

Dr. Sodhy seemed to be saying that he saw no reason why the women of Malaysia should make do with the "device" when the women of the United Kingdom and the United States preferred the Pill. "I wish to emphasize," he said, "that the illiterate and the poor are not necessarily unintelligent."

Intrauterine devices have been made available in Russia, but they are in short supply and only a few doctors have been trained in the technique of insertion. In India the family-planning experts originally thought the intrauterine device would answer, at least partially, the ever increasing birth rate, now skyrocketing at over a million per month. But the vast majority of women who attempted to use the Loop complained of excessive menstrual bleeding and pain. Planners then began to look for a better method.

The only other major form of contraception presently available is the Pill, the subject of this book. To see how it compares in effectiveness with other forms of contraception, examine the following table.

It may be seen from Table I that the sequential pills, one type of oral contraceptives, and IUD's are more than twice as effective as either the diaphragm or condom, perhaps the most commonly used contraceptives in this country. The combination pill, that is, the Pill, containing both estrogen and progestin—the bulk of the oral contraceptives now in use—has an effectiveness far exceeding any other method.

TABLE I

Method	Pregnancy Rate*
Douche	31
Rhythm	24
Jelly alone	20
Coitus Interruptus	18
Condom	14
Diaphragm	12
Intrauterine devices	5.0**
Sequential Pills } Oral Contraceptives	5.0***
Combination Pills	0.1****

* Number of pregnancies occurring if 100 women use the method for one year. This may also be stated as a percentage.[19]
** The latest report of the Advisory Committee on Obstetrics and Gynecology to the Federal Food and Drug Administration states, "The most successful IUD's are associated with a pregnancy rate of from 1.5 to 3.0 per 100 women during the first year of use. These rates tend to decline during successive years."
*** The higher incidence of pregnancies reported with the sequential pills is undoubtedly due to patient failure; omission of one or two pills permits ovulation to occur and since the anti-estrogenic effect of the progestin (in the combined variety) on cervical mucus and the lining of the uterus is not present, pregnancies occur more commonly.
**** This is a figure calculated to give every benefit to doubt. Actually, two large studies showed pregnancy rates of 0.028 and 0.023. Indeed, there are authorities who maintain that *every* pregnancy occurring among women using oral contraceptives has been the result of failure to take the Pill as directed.

In terms of theoretical effectiveness, the Pill provides 100 per cent protection against pregnancy, the IUD 98 per cent, and the diaphragm and condom 95 per cent or more. These late figures have been provided by the American College of Obstetricians and Gynecologists.[20] In actual practice, of course, the effectiveness of a contraceptive depends upon the patients as well as the method. Some women forget to take the Pill, some do not tolerate the heavier periods with an IUD, some dislike the untidiness of a diaphragm and jelly, and some object to the diminished sensation associated with the condom. Therefore, the choice of a method must be made on the basis of patient preference, as well as clinical performance.

In the next chapter, the reason for the extraordinary effectiveness of the Pill will be discussed.

3. How the Pill Works

I F ONE DESIRED to develop a contraceptive that was 100 per cent effective, an obvious way would be to prevent ovulation. This is exactly what the Pill does, and, perhaps surprisingly, by a rather simple process. That statement makes use of a great deal of hindsight, for when research began, knowledge about the hormones of pregnancy was meager. It had to be learned with effort and expense. But to understand the simple way in which the Pill works, we must take advantage of hindsight.

A woman is born with about a half million eggs in her ovaries. During her lifetime, however, she uses only about four hundred. Each egg, microscopic in size, is contained in a follicle, a miniature droplet containing a small amount of fluid.

The process of ovulation (egg release) begins when the ovaries secrete a small amount of estrogen. This hormone travels through the blood to a portion of the brain known as the *hypothalamus*. This most important area regulates most of the involuntary body functions, but it is particularly geared to the control of the endocrine system. Reaching this area, estrogen stimulates the hypothalamus to secrete a substance with the cumbersome name of

Follicle Stimulating Hormone Releasing Factor—FSH-RF. But the term describes exactly what happens.

The Releasing Factor, also a hormone, acts as a chemical signal to the pituitary gland. The pituitary is the major control gland of all other endocrine glands. It dispatches hormones through the blood to regulate the thyroid, the adrenals, and the ovaries. The word pituitary means "maker of mucus" in Latin, a misleading name given to it by seventeenth-century anatomists who incorrectly believed the gland to be the source of nasal mucus. The pituitary is about the size of a small lima bean and lies beneath the brain in a crevice in the skull called the *sella turcica*, or "Turk's saddle," a very descriptive term for the shape of the skull in this area.

Upon signal from the hypothalamus, the pituitary releases *Follicle Stimulating Hormone*—FSH. This, as the name suggests, stimulates the tiny follicles containing the eggs to grow and ripen until they appear as transparent bubbles on the surface of the ovary. At this point, another chemical signal is released from the ovaries. Its exact nature is unknown, but it is probably a form of estrogen. This hormone stimulates the hypothalamus to secrete *Luteinizing Hormone Releasing Factor*—LH-RF. This hormone is transmitted to the pituitary as a chemical messenger causing the release of *Luteinizing Hormone*—LH.

Why is only one follicle brought to the surface and prepared for ovulation each month? Again, the exact mechanism is unknown, but it is known that small amounts of estrogen stimulate the release of hormones from the hypothalamus, whereas large amounts prevent the release. As the major follicle is growing, it produces estrogen in its own cells. As the follicle becomes larger and larger, it secretes more estrogen. Thus, the follicle itself preserves its dominance since the estrogen it secretes gradually causes the amount of FSH to diminish, and other follicles stop growing and the eggs are destroyed. This happens each month and accounts for the discrepancy between the number of eggs provided and the number used in ovulation.

To return to LH, this hormone has two functions. First, it causes rupture of the most mature follicle, thus releasing the egg. Second, it is necessary for the production of *progesterone,* the hormone necessary for the establishment and continuation of pregnancy. This may be better understood if the sequential pattern by which the ovary produces its hormones is known. The ovary starts with *cholesterol,* a fatty substance that is the building block for all hormones. By using its own enzymes, the ovary converts cholesterol into an intermediate compound, *pregneneolone,* which in turn is converted into *progesterone.* Progesterone is changed into *androstenedione* (a male hormone also made in the testes!) and then finally to *estrogen.* It is obvious that one of the basic differences between man and woman is the fact that her ovaries contain an extra enzyme capable of changing male hormone into female hormone. Where does LH fit into this scheme? LH is able to change the cell structure in the ruptured follicle so that an abundance of progesterone (the third step in the production of estrogen), as well as estrogen, is produced and released.

After ovulation, the mass of cells in the ruptured follicle assumes a yellow tinge, probably due to the deposition of certain fat-laden cells from which both estrogen and progesterone are being released. This yellow body, known as the corpus luteum, is formed within twenty-four hours of ovulation and persists for about ten days in the normal menstrual cycle. Just as the follicle is stimulated to grow by FSH, the corpus luteum is stimulated by LH. And, just as FSH is gradually diminished by estrogen, LH is gradually diminished by progesterone. This is a process known as a "negative feedback," that is, as more hormone is made by the ovary, less ovarian stimulating hormone is released by the pituitary. What causes the demise of the corpus luteum? Its own hormone, progesterone.

For about ten days, that is, up until the twenty-third or twenty-fourth day of a twenty-eight-day cycle, progesterone is secreted in large amounts. Then, as the amount of LH is diminished, the corpus luteum begins to degenerate and the amounts of estrogen and progesterone are markedly reduced. The net result is an inadequate amount of hormones to maintain the lining of the womb. The tissue degenerates, blood vessels crumble, and menstruation occurs.

The large amounts of estrogen and progesterone produced by the yellow body have other very important functions. Estrogen prepares the breasts so that, in pregnancy, the high levels of progesterone effectively change the cells so that milk may be formed. Estrogen also thickens the lining of the uterus so that it becomes receptive to the fertilized egg. It does this by stimulating the blood vessels and the glands of the endometrium to increase in size and number.

Progesterone is needed to prepare the endometrium so that, on the sixth or seventh day after ovulation, the fertilized egg will find it easy to implant. Progesterone should be considered the "pregnancy hormone," for that is precisely what the term means. Progesterone is derived from two Latin words Pro and Gestare, meaning, "in favor of pregnancy." What does the hormone do that makes it so important? First, it strengthens the stroma of the endometrium, a lattice-like tissue that supports both the blood vessels and the glands. Thus, a firmer area for implantation is produced. Secondly, it depresses the constant, rhythmic muscular contractions of the uterus so that the egg, once implanted, will not be dislodged. But of even more importance, progesterone stimulates the glands of the endometrium to release a simple sugar called glycogen, a necessary food for sustenance of the new life present in the uterus.

If implantation occurs, the yellow body continues to function for forty to forty-five days. Eventually, other hormonal changes occur which force the placenta, the sac in which the fetus dwells, to produce estrogen and progesterone, and the yellow body dwindles to a scar on the surface of the ovary. If implantation does not occur, the thickened endometrium is discarded by menstruation, and a new cycle in preparation for pregnancy begins. Menstruation, then, is simply the process by which the body rids itself of tissue needed for pregnancy. It serves no useful purpose and is not necessary for health.

I promised that with hindsight it would be simple to see how the Pill works. The Pill contains quantities of estrogen and a progestin, which is a synthetic form of progesterone, in amounts sufficient to duplicate the actions of the body's natural hormones

—and to diminish release of FSH and LH. With low FSH, there is no development of the follicle containing the egg. With low LH, there is no rupture of the follicle. This is the principle. In actual practice, the progestin eliminates the surge of LH needed to rupture the follicle. The estrogen in the Pill, however, permits production of a small amount of FSH. The follicles grow a little, but never approach maturity.

One of the important questions to be asked is whether the Pill, since it acts upon the pituitary, affects control of the "master gland" over the adrenal and thyroid. Does the Pill "upset" the whole endocrine system? Extensive and prolonged investigation has led to an unequivocal answer: No. The Pill has no effect on adrenal or thyroid *function*. Estrogen does affect thyroid and adrenal hormones in the blood by the same method that occurs during pregnancy. More of each hormone attaches itself to blood proteins and, if this is measured, an elevated level is obtained. This does not mean, however, that the function of these glands has been altered by estrogen.

Another logical question might be: why combine estrogen and progestin in the Pill when either one can suppress ovulation? This question is perhaps best answered by removing the hindsight and going back to some of the problems that confronted the researchers who developed the Pill.

THE DEVELOPMENT OF THE PILL

In the winter of 1950, a physician, a biologist, and a nurse met in a New York City apartment to discuss the possibility of creating an ideal contraceptive agent. The physician was Dr. Abraham Stone who, with his wife, Dr. Hannah Stone, had pioneered in the development of the world's first clinic for infertile couples. The biologist was Dr. Gregory Pincus, then codirector of the Worcester Foundation for Experimental Biology in Shrewsbury, Massachusetts. The nurse was Margaret Sanger, founder of the Planned Parenthood movement. Abraham Stone read an item from an old medical journal to his guests that stated, "The ideal contraceptive still remains to be developed. It should be harmless, entirely reli-

able, simple, practical, universally applicable, and aesthetically
satisfactory to both husband and wife." Abraham and Hannah
Stone had written that description fifteen years previously.[21]

Stone explained that the research committee of the Planned
Parenthood Federation had allocated most of their funds to the
improvement of present methods, that is, diaphragms and spermi-
cides. But, he said, the Federation would endeavor to put up the
money if Pincus would "provide the brains and time" so that a
better contraceptive might be developed.

The amount of money donated by the Planned Parenthood Research Fund was only $2,100, scarcely enough to pay for the ani-
mals Pincus needed to initiate his experiments. To finance the
work properly, an additional $20,000 to $30,000 had to be raised.
But work was begun. Pincus, together with his codirector, Hudson
Hoagland, and his senior scientist, Min-Chueh Chang, formulated
an experimental design which they hoped might lead to an effective and safe oral contraceptive.

Among the "tools" used by Pincus and his associates in his animal
experimentation were estrogen and progesterone, and imperfect
tools they were. Estrogenic substances were available to the physician during the 1930's, but they were not widely accepted nor
extensively used. The skepticism of the medical profession was
intensified by a report by Professor Lacassagne of France, stating
that he had produced breast cancer in mice by administration of
estrogens. Furthermore, in those days estrogens were both weak
in potency and variable in effect, and had to be injected to obtain
demonstrable results. Since estrogenic substances, given by injection at repeated intervals, had a cumulative effect, they produced
excessive uterine bleeding, a most unwanted side effect.

Unfortunately, the "magic female hormone"—estrogen—became a tool of the quack, who used it to dupe women with fading
femininity and to enrich his own pockets. Patients were given estrogens by injection on a regular schedule, not by demonstrated need.
A nurse usually administered the "shot" so that the patient rarely
saw the physician. Even worse, she rarely had a thorough physical
examination. If the unscrupulous physician wished to improve the
waning sex drive of his patient, he simply added a small amount

of male hormone to the injection. While this male stimulus might have assisted a few individuals by increasing libido, the majority were unimproved. Rather, they developed undesirable side effects of acne, facial-hair growth, and deepening of the voice.

It is little wonder, then, that estrogen was looked upon with suspicion by the medical profession and that purveyors of the drug were considered charlatans.

As estrogenic substances became increasingly purified and their potency increased, their acceptance into medical practice was rapid. In the 1940's, synthetic estrogenic substances became available, and both these and natural hormones were used for treatment of many female disorders. Among these were premature menopause, premenopausal symptoms, congenital absence of the ovaries, removal of the ovaries during hysterectomy, painful menstruation, endometriosis, habitual abortion, and even the management of metastatic cancer of the breast in the postmenopausal female. Almost thirty years later, physicians are still using estrogens for the same disorders, and thousands of patients have taken them for over twenty-five years.

As useful as estrogen was in the 1940's, it was not an unmixed blessing. Problems resulted from its use. A major side effect was weight gain, but this might have been expected. Estrogen is a protein anabolic substance, that is, it aids metabolism of protein in muscular tissue. Furthermore, it causes retention of salt and water in body tissue, resulting in bloating and edema. Estrogen also affects the breasts, stimulating the growth of glandular cells, the ducts, and supporting tissues. Enlarged and painful breasts may occur in overly sensitive women. But the most serious problem was the effect of the hormone on the lining of the uterus, the endometrium. Here, estrogen stimulates growth of glands, supporting tissue (stroma), and blood vessels. Thus a woman taking estrogen may develop profuse and irregular bleeding. Estrogen, if administered constantly, may produce an overgrowth of the uterine lining called hyperplasia, which is considered to be a precursor of cancer in overly sensitive or predisposed women.

As Pincus worked with estrogen to suppress ovulation in animals, he discovered it was not always 100 per cent effective. Occasionally the pituitary would override the estrogenic suppression and release FSH and LH anyway, permitting ovulation and pregnancy.

Progesterone was available to Pincus, but it had many deficiencies. In the first place, progesterone had to be obtained from animal sources, the corpus luteum of the sow. It took thousands of ovaries to make 100 milligrams (mgs) of progesterone and, in order to suppress ovulation in the human, at least 300 mgs. had to be taken daily by mouth. Compare this to estrogen—only 0.1 mg. being needed to produce the same effect. Obviously, estrogen is a much more potent substance and more applicable in the formulation of a contraceptive pill. Secondly, the cost of progesterone as an oral medication was prohibitive. It became obvious that a combination of the potent hormone, estrogen, and the less potent but important hormone, progesterone, was necessary. After all, was this not a duplication of pregnancy—elevated estrogen and progesterone? Unfortunately, only a weak synthetic progesterone-like compound, a progestin called Pranone, was available to Pincus. This compound was a variation of the male hormone testosterone that had been altered by biochemists of the German Schering Corp. It is exactly the same as the progestins in use today except for a minor alteration in its structure.

As Pincus labored in his Shrewsbury laboratory, another development was occurring at the Free Hospital for Women (now the Boston Hospital for Women) in Brookline, Massachusetts, where Dr. John Rock was attempting to relieve sterility in women in whom no specific cause for their barrenness could be found. Rock observed that in a number of patients the tubes and the uterus were tiny and underdeveloped. One of Dr. Rock's young research fellows, Dr. Herbert W. "Trader" Horne, suggested that this deficiency might be corrected by creating a pseudopregnancy if both estrogen and progesterone were given constantly and for prolonged periods of time. Rock gathered eighty women, all of whom had been infertile for two to six years. Then he administered increasingly large doses of a synthetic estrogen known as DES (diethylstilbestrol), plus similarly increasingly large doses of progesterone. For three months these eighty patients were hormonally pregnant, and many noted symptoms of normal pregnancy. They complained of nausea, tenderness and enlargement of the breasts, as well as increased pigmentation of the nipples. After the "pseudo-pregnancy" was over, thirteen of the patients became pregnant. Rock felt this was an improvement over what could be expected by chance alone.

At this time, 1951, Rock and Pincus met at a scientific conference and exchanged details of their experiments. At the suggestion of Pincus, Rock designed a new clinical experiment using progesterone alone. Rather than administer it constantly, he planned to give it from the fifth to the twenty-fifth day of the ovarian cycle, then withdraw the drug to permit menstruation.

Rock gathered another twenty-seven women, all of whom had been infertile for more than two years. When these patients took only progesterone in twenty-day cycles, most tests showed that ovulation had ceased. Furthermore, the undesirable symptoms associated with pseudopregnancy did not occur. This new and less emotionally disturbing regimen resulted in subsequent pregnancy in four of the twenty-seven patients who completed at least three months of artificial cycles.

This experiment proved to Pincus that progesterone, if given in adequate amounts, could inhibit ovulation in humans as well as in laboratory animals; but both Pincus and Rock were disappointed with the performance of natural progesterone. Almost 20 per cent of the patients developed "breakthrough" bleeding during the time they were taking the pill. Although this could be overcome easily by a prompt increase in dosage, the bleeding was disturbing to most patients. Another important observation indicated that progesterone inhibited ovulation only about 85 per cent of the time. This appeared to be a major drawback to its use as an oral contraceptive. Of even greater importance, tremendous doses of progesterone were required to suppress ovulation when administered orally.

It was obvious, then, that a compound as harmless as progesterone, but with increased potency, was urgently needed. The compound would have to be inexpensive and capable of preventing ovulation in every cycle. It should result in a normal flow and not cause irregular bleeding. In the fall of 1953, Pincus asked several pharmaceutical companies to supply him with samples of all progesterone-like substances that their chemists had synthesized.

It was fortunate that in the early 1950's, the G. D. Searle Co. and Syntex Laboratory had begun independent research programs to develop new oral substances that had the properties of progesterone. In the laboratories of G. D. Searle, the aim was to develop an oral progestin for treatment of menstrual disorders—and an oral contraceptive. A group of chemists under Dr. Byron Reigel began a search for suitable compounds.

One of the chemists in the group was Dr. Frank Colton, formerly of the Mayo Clinic and an assistant in that institution to Dr. Edward C. Kendall, who developed cortisone. Colton concentrated his efforts on the synthesis of what were called "19-norsteroids." These had properties similar to progesterone but chemically were quite different. They were really much more like the male hormone testosterone. But chemists have amazing ingenuity, and the chemists at G. D. Searle were no exception. They found that if *one* carbon atom (with its usual complement of three attached hydrogen atoms) was removed from the old compound Pranone, a much more potent compound with properties like progesterone resulted. The term "19-nor" simply means that this carbon was removed at the nineteenth position in the structure. Furthermore, by rearranging the molecular structure, they were able to make a *testosterone-like* compound *estrogen-like*. The result? A substance with the properties of naturally occurring progesterone but with only eighteen instead of the twenty-one carbon atoms needed in progesterone. Thus the term *progestin*. Furthermore, these substances were very much like male hormone but devirilized by removal of one carbon atom. What could be better? A variant of a male hormone, but really feminine, that had the effects of progesterone. And a bonus—it was effective orally!

The first "19-norprogestin" had been synthesized by Professor Maximillian Ehrenstein at the University of Pennsylvania in 1945, but Prof. Ehrenstein was interested in finding a compound that would stimulate heart function. Although he found his "19-norprogestin" ineffective for this purpose, he described it as having an effect similar to that of progesterone.

In the summer of 1952, Colton devised the synthesis of an entire new series of 19-norsteroids. One of these had an exceptionally high score when tested in animals; moreover, it was nontoxic in humans! This compound was given the identification number SC-4642 and the generic name *norethynodrel*. In animal studies it was found to have a marked progestational effect.

When Pincus asked G. D. Searle for samples of a progesterone-like substance, he was forwarded a sample of SC-4642. By the end of 1954, he had completed the animal investigation and realized that this drug was sufficiently potent to be effective in suppressing ovulation in women. A small sample of the compound was submitted to Rock and his associates for clinical studies.

Fifty infertile women were recruited for a third series of tests. Each woman was observed for a month to make certain of ovulation, then each began taking SC-4642 orally from the fifth through the twenty-fourth day of her cycle. Whereas the natural progesterone had been administered in doses of 300 mgs. daily, the SC-4642 was given in much smaller amounts, some receiving 50 mgs. daily, others as little as 10 mgs.

Despite the smaller doses, the new compound suppressed ovulation in virtually 100 per cent of the patients. In the months subsequent to testing, six of the previously infertile women became pregnant.

Pincus and Rock realized that the new 19-norsteroids, particularly norethynodrel, were far more active in inhibiting ovulation and produced far fewer side effects than the natural progesterone-plus-estrogen used earlier. Rock was particularly pleased that some of his patients became pregnant after taking the drug. His principal interest, after all, was in treating infertility, not in developing an oral contraceptive.

Five years had elapsed since Gregory Pincus began his search for an oral contraceptive with an idea, optimism, and a grant of $2,100. During those five years, many unpredicted problems had arisen, necessitating a collaboration among chemists, biologists, and physicians. The cost was not $2,100, but well over $300,000.

Unknown to Pincus and Rock, there was a large element of chance involved in their work. Their idea was to suppress ovulation by the use of a progestin alone. It would not, they believed, have the undesirable side effects of estrogen, such as weight gain, painful breasts, and excessive menstruation. When SC-4642 was first available, it contained a small amount of estrogen. This was a "contaminant" remaining from the method of production. Neither Pincus nor Rock wanted this estrogen. They wanted a pure progestin. With efforts, chemists at G. D. Searle managed to remove the estrogen. To the surprise of everyone, the pure progestin was not as effective. Too many patients developed breakthrough bleeding. When the "contaminating" estrogen was deliberately re-added to the progestin, breakthrough bleeding was minimal. This should have been anticipated; estrogen is the "building block" of the endometrium. It prevents its degeneration. Ultimately, the "contaminated" SC-4642 was marketed as the Pill, Enovid, which initially contained 9.85 mgs. of *norethynodrel* and 0.15 mg. of an estrogen known as *mestranol*.

There is another aspect to the story of the development of the Pill: my interest in finding improved methods of treating endometriosis. This disease occurs when portions of the endometrium escape from the open ends of the Fallopian tubes during menstruation. This living tissue clings to the ovaries, tubes, intestines, and other organs in the pelvic region. The errant tissue continues to grow, to bleed each month just like the endometrium lining the uterus, and eventually to alter the function of the ovary. Consider these minute areas of misplaced tissue as hundreds of little wombs, each menstruating every month, but unlike the parent endometrium, this tissue is confined under the tender lining of the pelvis, the peritoneum. Each month the bleeding area distends the peritoneum over it, irritates the nerve fibers, and gradually spreads. Month after month, year after year (unless menstruation is stopped by menopause or pregnancy) the peritoneum is insulted by more menstrual blood from the tubes. No wonder the disease is associated with painful menstruation!

Endometriosis is one of the major causes of infertility. The misplaced tissue, bleeding as it does each month, produces extensive scar tissue and adhesions around the Fallopian tubes and ovaries. Although the tubes remain open, they become tangled in the web of adhesions and cannot move. When the egg is released from the ovary, the open end of the tube just cannot grasp it. Infertility is further encouraged by the fact that intercourse becomes so painful it is practically impossible to provide adequate sperm at the optimum time.

Among my patients in 1956 was a nurse who suffered from a severe case of endometriosis. By a stroke of remarkable good fortune, she managed to become pregnant, despite the obstacles, and progressed uneventfully to her due date. At that time, because of a small pelvis and a breech presentation of the baby, it was necessary to deliver her by Caesarian section. During surgery I saw that her endometriosis had disappeared. All that remained was some brown, crumbly material around the tubes and ovaries. Our pathologist reported it to be dead endometrial tissue.

It has long been axiomatic among gynecologists that the best treatment for endometriosis is pregnancy. Nine months without menstruation permits some degree of healing to occur. The trouble is that endometriosis makes it difficult to become pregnant. It had been suspected for some time that the reason pregnancy had such a salutary effect on endometriosis was that the placenta produced such large amounts of estrogen. The estrogen caused softening of the endometriosis and the absence of menstruation prevented further "seeding." The usual treatment for endometriosis prior to 1957 was to give estrogen in very large doses. Although effective, this method produced undesirable side effects: weight gain, bloating, and recurrent bleeding. I remember doing repeated curettages on women receiving excessive doses of estrogen for endometriosis. The tissue I curetted from the uterus had been overstimulated, the glands became "hyperplastic," and the blood vessels enlarged and congested.

Other investigators had used male hormone, testosterone, to control the symptoms of endometriosis, but, all too frequently, patients complained of acne, oily skin, and excessive hair growth.

It seemed logical to me to attempt to treat endometriosis with a combination of estrogen and progesterone, just like pregnancy, but in the early 1950's no such product was available. I went to the William S. Merrell Co. in Cincinnati to ask if they had a progesterone-like drug that they could add to the estrogen they already marketed. The director of clinical research said he could anticipate "no market for such a drug in the foreseeable future." This has to rank as one of the least prophetic statements ever made.

During this time I frequently attended conferences held by Dr. Rock at his fertility clinic. During one of the meetings, he mentioned the drug SC-4642. It sounded ideal for my experiments. Dr. William J. Crosson, then director of clinical investigation for G. D. Searle, promptly sent me a supply, and I devised a plan of treatment that simulated the hormonal changes of pregnancy. Most fortunately, the drug I received was the "contaminated" progestin —perfect for my purposes. Its use on patients with endometriosis had a most therapeutic effect.

The question that led to this discussion of the history of the development of the Pill was: Why use both estrogen and progestin when either one suppresses ovulation? The progestin has several effects when combined with estrogen. First, it potentiates the effect of estrogen because both suppress the functions of the pituitary. Thus, the occasional escape of the pituitary from estrogen suppression is prevented by the progestin. Rarely, if ever, does ovulation occur. But, even if it does, the progestin has other important effects which, acting alone, are capable of preventing conception. How? By its remarkable anti-estrogenic property that is exerted on both the endometrium and the cervical mucus. Progestin changes the endometrium so that it is "out of phase," making implantation of the fertilized egg impossible.

Secondly, the progestin negates the effect of estrogen on cervical mucus so that sperm cannot penetrate. Their migration into the uterus is prevented just as it is after ovulation. Thus the Pill works in three ways, suppressing ovulation, preventing implantation, and changing cervical mucus so that it is unreceptive to sperm. A bonus is added since the progestin prevents the overgrowth of the endometrium, permitting a more normal and often scantier flow.

With some hindsight again, it may seem strange that there was any doubt that the Pill, as developed in 1955 and 1956, would work. But it was entirely appropriate that five years of clinical testing be required before it won approval for public use by the Federal Food and Drug Administration. The testing was performed by many clinicians, but the principal study was done in Puerto Rico under Dr. Celso Ramon Garcia. Puerto Rico was selected because it has one of the highest pregnancy rates in the world and because Pincus and Rock were eager to know if unsophisticated women were able to follow directions for taking the medication.

The study has been on-going in Puerto Rico since 1956. Two oral contraceptives have been used, Enovid and Ovulen, both made by G. D. Searle. Enovid has been used by 811 women for a total of 25,063 cycles, and Ovulen by 497 women for 11,452 cycles. There are, thus, women who have been observed while taking the Pill for twelve years. Not only has the medication been virtually 100 per cent effective as a contraceptive, but, as a recent report on the study states, "It is impressive that there have been no cases of thrombophlebitis, cardiovascular accidents (strokes), coronaries, diabetes, or other morbidities of a significant nature occurring among the long-term contraceptive users in this study."[22]

4. Brands of Pills and How to Use Them

THEY ARE SMALL, these pills, no larger than an ordinary aspirin tablet. They come in all colors, white, blue, yellow, and pink. Actually, they should be called tablets—since pills are spherical and these are flat. They are hormones with unusual potency. But, most important, they are being swallowed by the billions. They have lighted the fuse of revolutions in medicine, sociology, theology, and sexual behavior.

The Pill that was first used in 1956, tested in Puerto Rico, then approved for public use in 1961, is now largely a museum piece. The G. D. Searle Co. still markets the original Pill, but its use is restricted to treatment of menstrual or other female disorders. No knowledgeable physician would prescribe it for contraceptive purposes alone. *That* pill is no longer *the* Pill, for, through the years, investigation showed that much, much smaller doses of both progestin and estrogen effectively prevent ovulation. This was all to the good, since side effects are directly related to the amount of hormone in the Pill.

At this writing, there are twenty-two brands of the Pill marketed in the United States, each differing in the type and dosage of its component hormones.* Sixteen of the brands are called "combination" pills, that is, each tablet contains both progestin and estrogen. Four brands are called "sequentials." The first fourteen to sixteen pills contain only estrogen, while the last five or six pills contain a combination of progestin and estrogen. Table II identifies the brands and dosages.

The array of oral contraceptives shown in Table II (and more are likely to be marketed soon) reflects the competitive spirit of the pharmaceutical industry. Not only has competition lowered the price, the constant search by chemists has resulted in more potent agents which produce the desired effect with a minimum of side effects. The multiplicity of brands has important advantages to both the physician and the patient. With the exception of Ortho-Novum and Norinyl, each brand is different, making it possible to tailor the prescription to fit the peculiar needs of each patient.

THE DIFFERENCES BETWEEN BRANDS

One of the differences between the brands of pills, as Table II shows, is in the amount of progestin and estrogen they contain. Rock and Pincus originally believed that progestin alone suppressed ovulation; therefore a large amount of it was needed. Thus the original Pill (Enovid 10) contained 9.85 mgs. of progestin and .15 mg. of estrogen. As investigation continued, it became obvious that lesser amounts of progestin could be used if the amount of estrogen was kept fairly constant. By 1961, when the Pill won FDA approval, Enovid was marketed with only 5 mgs. of progestin. Three years later, Enovid-E was released. The amount of progestin was reduced to 2.5 mgs. and estrogen increased from .075 to 0.1 mg. The effectiveness of the Pill was unchanged, but the incidence of side effects was markedly reduced.

It is now known that ovulation can be suppressed with as little as .075 mg. to .08 mg. (or 75 to 80 micrograms) of estrogen. Yet, the combination pills, Norinyl-1, Norlestrin, Norlestrin-1, Ortho-Novum-1, Provest, and Ovral are marketed with only .05 mg. of

* An exception: Ortho-Novum and Norinyl are identical.

TABLE II

Oral Contraceptives in the United States

TRADEMARK	MANUFACTURER	TYPE	PROGESTOGEN	PROGESTOGEN MG/TAB	ESTROGEN	ESTROGEN MG/TAB	TOTAL STEROIDS MG/TAB
Enovid 10 mg.	Searle	Comb.	norethynodrel	9.85	mestranol	.15	10.00
Enovid 5 mg.	Searle	Comb.	norethynodrel	5.0	mestranol	.075	5.075
Ortho-Novum 10 mg.	Ortho	Comb.	norethindrone	10.0	mestranol	.06	10.06
Ortho-Novum 2 mg.	Ortho	Comb.	norethindrone	2.0	mestranol	.10	2.10
Enovid-E	Searle	Comb.	norethynodrel	2.5	mestranol	.10	2.60
Norlestrin 2.5 mg.	Parke-Davis	Comb.	norethindrone acetate	2.5	ethinyl estradiol	.05	2.55
Norinyl	Syntex	Comb.	norethindrone	2.0	mestranol	.10	2.10
Provest	Upjohn	Comb.	medroxyprogesterone	10.0	ethinyl estradiol	.05	10.05
C-Quens	Eli Lilly	Seq.	chlormadinone acetate	2.0	mestranol	.08	2.08
Oracon	Mead Johnson	Seq.	dimethisterone	25.0	ethinyl estradiol	.10	25.10
Ovulen	Searle	Comb.	ethynodiol diacetate	1.0	mestranol	.10	1.10
Ovulen-21	Searle	Comb.	ethynodiol diacetate	1.0	mestranol	.10	1.10
Ovulen-28	Searle	Comb.	ethynodiol diacetate	1.0	mestranol	.10	1.10
Ortho-Novum SQ	Ortho	Seq.	norethindrone	2.0	mestranol	.08	2.08
Ortho-Novum 1 mg.	Ortho	Comb.	norethindrone	1.0	mestranol	.05	1.05
Ortho-Novum 1-80	Ortho	Comb.	norethindrone	1.0	mestranol	.08	1.08
Norinyl-1	Syntex	Comb.	norethindrone	1.0	mestranol	.05	1.05
Norlestrin 1 mg.	Parke-Davis	Comb.	norethindrone acetate	1.0	ethinyl estradiol	.05	1.05
Norlestrin 28-1	Parke-Davis	Comb.	norethindrone acetate	1.0	ethinyl estradiol	.05	1.05
Norquen	Syntex	Seq.	norethindrone	2.0	mestranol	.08	2.08
Noriday	Syntex	Comb.	norethindrone	1.0	mestranol	.05	1.05
Ovral®	Wyeth	Comb.	norgestrel	.5	ethinyl estradiol	.05	.55

estrogen. Recently the amount of estrogen in Ortho-Novum-1 was increased to .08 mg. In these preparations, the potent progestin aids and abets the lower dose of estrogen in suppressing the pituitary and prevents ovulation. The amount of progestin in these "mini-dose" pills varies from 10 mg. in Provest (a weak progestin) to .50 mg. in Ovral (a potent progestin). Certain side effects are estrogen induced (nausea, bloating) and therefore attempts have been made to include the minimal amount of this hormone. But, if the estrogen level is too low, another side effect, *breakthrough bleeding*, occurs. This is an individual problem. Some women never have bleeding or spotting while taking preparations with only .05 mg. of estrogen, whereas others always do. In some instances, the endometrium will adapt to the low estrogen and bleeding ceases after three or four cycles. But certain women find it necessary to take pills containing .1 mg. of estrogen and, for them, Norinyl-2, Ortho-Novum-2, Enovid-E or Ovulen must be prescribed. I have a few patients, inclined to clinical investigation, who find that they are able to avoid the bloating and nausea, and the bleeding, if they take Norinyl-1, Ortho-Novum-1, or Norlestrin-1 during the first ten days, then double the dose during the last ten days. This is perfectly satisfactory, but I warn them never to do the opposite! If the pituitary is held in check by .1 mg. of estrogen and then the dose is abruptly reduced to half that, a burst of LH is released and ovulation occurs. Of course, they have the added protection of the action of the progestin on the endometrium and cervical mucus, but why take chances?

The other major difference between the brands reflects the characteristics of the particular types of estrogen and, particularly, progestin they contain. All of the brands of combination pills use one of two types of estrogen, either mestranol or ethinyl estradiol. They are essentially the same compound but mestranol has the advantage of lasting a little longer and the disadvantage of having more side effects. Remember that estradiol is the estrogen produced in the human ovary. The most widely publicized estrogen is sodium estrone sulfate, marketed as Premarin, and extracted from the urine of pregnant mares. It is a naturally occurring estrogen—estrone is also made in the human ovary—whereas mestranol and ethinyl estradiol are synthetically produced. Premarin has a minimum of side effects, but it is much too expensive to be incorporated in the Pill. The most commonly used estrogen in the world is DES (diethylstilbestrol). This synthetic compound is relatively inexpensive, but nausea and queasiness occur frequently, particularly at higher dosages. DES is one-tenth as potent as mestranol or ethinyl estradiol. Dosage, therefore, is ten times as great.

But it is really the progestin that accounts for the major differences between brands. There are three major types of synthetic progestin in use, one similar to progesterone; one similar to testosterone (male hormone); and one similar to estrogen. The most commonly used progestin is *norethindrone*, found in Norinyl, Norlestrin, Ortho-Novum, Norquen, and Ovral.* It is called an *androgenic* progestin because it tends to have more male side effects such as acne, increased hair growth, and accentuated libido. This progestin is also more protein anabolic, that is, it may increase appetite and consumption of calories, and it may increase the deposition of protein in muscular tissue, which, in certain patients, is of definite advantage. This is not to say that women taking this progestin will develop bulging muscles.

In my practice I prescribe one of the pills using norethindrone in patients who appear overly estrogenic. This individual frequently has large breasts that become extremely tender during the week prior to menstruation. I also select this progestin for women who are underweight and have scrawny muscular development. The effect on sex drive is variable, but occasionally subjective improvement is noted.

The second type of progestin is *norethynodrel*, the progestin which was, and still is, used in the original Pill, Enovid. Norethynodrel may be described as an *estrogenic* progestin, that is, it produces more feminizing side effects. It may cause breast enlargement both by stimulating cell growth and by increasing salt and water retention. It is important to remember that the net effect of two hormones on an organ such as the breast or uterus is depend-

---

* The norethindrone in Ovral is modified by the addition of one carbon and two hydrogen atoms, thus increasing the potency and changing its generic name to norgestrel.

ent on their similarity. Norethindrone, being only slightly estrogenic and basically androgenic, negates much of the estrogenic effect of the estrogen contained in the Pill. This accounts for the scanty flow and improvement in breast tenderness noted by many women. In Enovid, however, the estrogen in the Pill is potentiated by the estrogenic properties of the progestin norethynodrel. In women overly sensitive to estrogen, the net effect is that of excessive estrogen stimulation—nausea, weight gain, water retention, bloating.

I prescribe Enovid for women who appear to lack feminine characteristics. They usually have small breasts, suffer from acne, are rather hirsute, and have a strong sex drive.* Their ovaries probably produce an excess of male hormone and diminished estrogen. Since acne and excessive hair growth are side effects of the male hormone testosterone, these patients frequently note marked improvement in these undesirable traits. Enovid is an ideal preparation for them; it suppresses the pituitary, the ovaries rest; the secretion of male hormone from the ovaries is diminished; the full effect of estrogen plus an estrogenic progestin is frequently so acceptable that many patients are loathe to discontinue the medication. They like their new found femininity.

There is one other estrogenic progestin, Lyndiol, but at the moment it is marketed only outside the United States.

A third type of progestin is found in Provest. Its chemical structure is almost the same as the progesterone found in the body. It may be described as being neuter in its masculinizing or feminizing effects. It also has the least side effects of any of the progestins, but since it is combined with only .05 mg. of estrogen, a great tendency to breakthrough bleeding is noted.

The multiplicity of brands permits the physician a number of options in dealing with side effects. If a woman is taking Enovid, for example, complains of sore breasts, prolonged nausea, a bloated sensation, or diminished interest in sexual intercourse, substitution of a male-type pill may alleviate her problem. Or, if she notes

---

* It is a strange phenomenon that the big-bosomed, ultra-feminine women who tend to become sex symbols often have less sex drive than the small breasted women with rather male characteristics.

excessive weight gain and acne while taking an androgenic progestin, she might do better on Enovid or Provest or perhaps a brand with smaller dosage. Thus, the physician may adjust the dose or substitute a different pill to fit the body type of each patient.

HOW THE PILLS ARE TAKEN

Most combination pills marketed in the United States call for the woman to take a pill for twenty consecutive days each menstrual cycle. Allowing two or three days for the flow to begin and restarting the Pill five days later, a twenty-eight-day cycle is established.

The patient is instructed to take the Pill daily starting on Day 5 of her cycle, Day 1 being the first day of menstruation. At the end of twenty (or twenty-one) days, she stops taking the Pill and menstruation usually begins within two or three days. She resumes taking the Pill five days after the onset of flow. Most brands are packaged with various aids to remind the user that she has taken the Pill and to simplify counting the days. Such packaging may be looked upon as insurance, for it has been shown that even illiterate women can follow the regimen.

The exceptions to the above are Ovulen 21, Ovral, Noriday, and Norlestrin-28-1. Whether it be "shopping day," "bridge day," or "housecleaning" day, a woman is accustomed to thinking in terms of days of the week rather than "cycle days." These four brands let her remember her natural way. Once established, her starting day is always the same day of the week, because it is fixed at three weeks on, one week off, and is independent of withdrawal flow. Noriday has an added feature, seven "blank" pills that contain no hormone and are taken immediately after the twenty-first Norinyl tablet. This eliminates counting. It is simply a pill a day. Norlestrin-28, and Ovulen-28, just released, are similar—each package contains twenty-one estrogen-progestin tablets and seven inert ones.

For most users, these directions are all they ever need to know. But problems arise occasionally that lead to questions. The major difficulties seem to be these:

1. Occasionally bleeding persists for five full days. This is of no

significance, since the length and amount of bleeding following use of the Pill depends on the estrogen and progestin composition of the brand being used. The Pill should be restarted on Day 5 despite continuing flow. Within a day or two bleeding will cease. If bleeding is excessive while the Pill is being taken, a uterine curettage is mandatory.

2. Sometimes withdrawal flow does not occur after completing the series of twenty or twenty-one pills. This is due to the anti-estrogenic effect of the progestin in the Pill on the endometrium and is of no significance. The absence of menstruation occurs rarely, perhaps in 1 or 2 per cent of patients. It is important that the Pill be restarted no later than seven days after completing the previous series. I actually tell my patients to restart pill taking *within five days* if no period occurs. If the delay exceeds seven days—regardless of whether withdrawal flow has occurred—the risk of ovulation and pregnancy is quite high. Conceptions have been reported as a result of this "patient error." *To be safe, resume taking the Pill within five days if no withdrawal flow occurs.*

3. From time to time, spotting or a slight brownish discharge is noted while taking the Pill. I instruct my patients to continue the Pill as directed, and the spotting usually disappears. If, however, breakthrough bleeding occurs, two courses of action are available. One is to discontinue the Pill, consider the bleeding as regular menstruation, and resume the medication five days later. If the breakthrough bleeding occurs late in the cycle, however, the dose of the Pill may be doubled throughout the rest of that cycle. During the next cycle, one tablet is again taken daily. If breakthrough bleeding occurs again, the dose is again doubled. Usually after four or five cycles, the nuisance of breakthrough bleeding disappears. If it does not, the patient should consult her physician. He may elect to substitute a pill containing a larger amount of estrogen. Persistent breakthrough bleeding is abnormal. It requires a diagnostic survey, possibly a curettage, to be certain that a polyp or fibroid is not the cause.

4. Another distressing situation is occasioned by forgetting to take a pill. It is important that a definite pattern of pill taking be established. Ideally, it should be taken at the same time every day. We are all creatures of habit and eventually a habit pattern be-

comes second nature. I usually recommend that my patients take the Pill with their evening meal. The nausea associated with the first or second cycle is much less likely to occur. Or, the Pill can be taken at bedtime or upon arising, but whenever, a regular plan should be established.

If a pill is forgotten, it should be taken as soon as remembered, the next morning if the evening pill has been skipped. The next pill is taken at the regular time, even if the interval between them is short. If a combination pill is being used, the risk of pregnancy from missing one pill is practically zero. However, this protection is not afforded to users of the sequential pills. It should be obvious that even with the combination pills, the risk of pregnancy increases with the number of pills missed. Numerous studies have shown that there is virtually no chance of pregnancy when the pills are taken as directed. If one to five pills are missed, the pregnancy rate rises to 7.2 per cent. If six to nineteen pills are missed, the pregnancy rate rises to 31.2 per cent. However, if two or three pills are missed on consecutive days, the sustained effort of the medication on the endometrium is lost and breakthrough bleeding may occur.

There are two other circumstances that deserve emphasis. I always warn my patients to avoid intercourse during the first week of the *first* treatment cycle since ovulation may occur during this time. Also, if the patient changes brands of pills, intercourse should be avoided during the first week of the first "new pill" cycle. Ovulation is particularly likely to occur if the shift is from an agent containing .1 mg. of estrogen to one having only .05 mg. The pituitary gland escapes from estrogen suppression during the first week of the diminished medication and ovulation may occur.

There are other questions that arise concerning how young or how old a person can be and safely take the Pill, as well as when and if a nursing mother may start the medication. These questions will be answered in the appropriate chapters in Part II.

SEQUENTIAL PILLS

The sequential pills were designed to mimic the natural hormonal sequence of the ovary. They are packaged so that estrogen alone is given during the first fourteen to sixteen days, followed by an estrogen-progestin combination pill during the last five or six days. However, if you recall that progesterone is secreted during the *last fourteen* days of the cycle, the mimicry may be said to be incomplete.

There are four brands of sequential pills marketed in this country and each is a bit different. Oracon consists of sixteen consecutive pills containing .1 mg. of the estrogen ethinyl estradiol, followed by five pills containing the same estrogen plus 25 mgs. of a weak progestin known as dimethisterone. The progestin is similar to norethindrone but is much less potent. C-Quens consists of fifteen consecutive pills containing .08 mg. of mestranol, followed by five pills containing the same amount of estrogen plus 2.0 mgs. of a potent progestin, chlormadinone. This progestin is very much like progesterone; it is not a "19-norsteroid," but several changes in its structure have given it unusual potency.

Ortho-Novum SQ is similar to C-Quens in that the first fourteen pills (C-Quens has fifteen) contain only .08 mg. of mestranol and the last six (C-Quens has five) combine the same amount of estrogen with 2 mgs. of norethindrone. There really is little difference between these two sequentials, and both were designed to reduce the problems associated with combined regimens. If these problems are due to the progestin, the idea is acceptable. But if the side effects are due to the estrogen, I have not seen an appreciable difference between Oracon with .1 mg. of estrogen and C-Quens or Ortho-Novum SQ with .08 mg. Furthermore, the low estrogen skirts dangerously near the minimum needed to suppress ovulation consistently. Norquen, the fourth brand of sequentials, is the same as Ortho-Novum SQ.

An innovation in sequential oral contraceptives, soon to be marketed, employs a more physiological approach. This preparation, known as Profem, employs a graduated estrogen scheme followed by an estrogen-progestin combination. The first Pill is taken on the *first* day of bleeding in the first cycle, but it contains only .025 mg. of estrogen. These are taken for seven days. For the next fourteen days the Pill contains .1 mg. of estrogen—adequate to suppress ovulation. The last seven pills contain .125 mg. of estrogen plus 10 mgs. of a progestin, Provera (the same progestin used in Provest). After Pill 28, Pill 1 is restarted and a flow ensues in two or three days. This prevents the low estrogen levels that may be responsible for certain symptoms (headache, flushes) in patients using twenty-day or twenty-one-day regimens.

The major difficulty associated with the use of sequential agents is that missing just one pill is an invitation to pregnancy. The amount of estrogen is so low in C-Quens and Ortho-Novum SQ that ovulation may occur shortly after the omission of a single pill. Even if the estrogen is taken, a sudden bout of gastroenteritis or vomiting may prevent complete absorption. In the combined pill, alteration of the endometrium and cervical mucus are protective factors, but these are lacking with the sequentials. The risk of missing a single pill was reflected in Table I where sequential pills were shown to have a 5 per cent pregnancy rate. Excluding "patient failures," the sequentials are said to equal the combined pills in efficacy. Unfortunately, patients do fail!

In my opinion, the sequential agents are most useful during the premenopausal period. In this age group the chances of becoming pregnant, even if a pill is omitted, are considerably reduced. In the woman who is 45 to 52 years of age, the sequentials have several advantages: estrogen alone for the first fourteen to sixteen days is of great benefit to women demonstrating signs and symptoms of estrogen insufficiency. The absence of the progestin and its anti-estrogenic effects is highly desirable, since the estrogen is unopposed. The sequentials produce regular bleeding episodes at an age when women tend to have irregular and profuse flow. Finally, the five days of progestin prevents hyperplasia of the endometrium, a common occurrence if ovulation is irregular or absent.

EFFECTIVENESS OF THE PILL

If any reader questions the effectiveness of the Pill as a contraceptive (and that is possible), let him be reassured by the results of these observations: Enovid is the oldest and therefore the most extensively studied. Only three pregnancies occurred among 14,840 women using it for over 116,000 cycles, a pregnancy rate of .028 per cent. Using Ortho-Novum-2 (2 mgs. of progestin, .1 mg. of estrogen), the pregnancy rate was .023 per cent. In Europe, Anovlar and Lyndiol have given a similar rate of effectiveness. Provest, Ovulen, Norlestrin, and Norinyl have demonstrated an equivalent degree of efficacy, although the total number of patients studied is not of the same magnitude.

An advisory committee, headed by Dr. Louis M. Hellman, recently reported to the Federal Food and Drug Administration on the efficacy of the Pill. They concluded, "Even when oral contraception failures are considered to represent drug failures rather than patient failure in proper administration of the drug, these compounds are almost invariably effective."

II

EFFECTS OF
THE PILL

5. The Pill and Your Figure

ONE OF the phenomena of these times is the figure consciousness of women and the men who observe them. Fashions, notably the bikini and the miniskirt, impose demands on the figure that often approach the impossible, for when a woman diets to slenderize her waist and hips, one of the first places she loses fat is in the breasts. Nevertheless, being slender is of great importance to women—as a gynecologist would state it—from prepuberty to long past menopause.

Because women are so conscious of their figures, anything that affects the figure takes on great significance. Does the Pill affect a woman's figure? The Pill can improve a woman's figure or lead to unwanted weight gain or have no effect at all. Of these, the latter is by far the most common.

I begin this section of the book dealing with the effects of the Pill with the figure problem because weight gain is the most common reason women stop taking the Pill. This was shown in the survey of physicians conducted by the American College of Obstetricians and Gynecologists.

A number of studies have shown that the incidence of weight

63

gain among users of the Pill varies from 14 to 50 per cent, depending upon the type of population surveyed and the brand of oral contraceptive used. The amount of weight gained varies. Some women gain one or two pounds by the second month. They then gain slowly, adding a total of five or six pounds during the first six months. A few women report larger weight gains, occasionally as much as twenty pounds. However, the majority of patients weigh within two pounds of their pre-pill weight at the end of a year of therapy.

It is difficult to evaluate the reasons for the weight gain. Some women just feel so much better while on the Pill that they develop an improved appetite. Alleviation of menstrual discomfort and the relief from fear of pregnancy often lead to a sense of well-being and increased caloric intake.

But the Pill itself has the side effect of causing weight gain for some, though certainly not all women. In most patients the added pounds are temporary, but a few maintain the extra weight until the Pill is stopped. The more androgenic progestins, particularly norethindrone, are associated with an increased formation of body tissue—but not fat. This was evident when the 10 mgs. dose of Ortho-Novum was marketed. About 50 per cent of the women taking this preparation gained weight. A smaller percentage of women report weight gain on the 2 mg. dose, and even less when only 1 mg. is used. The other brands using norethindrone (Norinyl, Norlestrin, Ovulen) have essentially the same tendency. The more estrogenic progestin in Enovid and the neutral progestins in Provest and C-Quens produce less permanent weight gain.

Temporary weight gain is the direct result of a physiological action of estrogen. This hormone prevents the usual excretion of salt (sodium chloride) by the kidneys and the retained salt attracts water to it. In medical terminology this is called edema. This happens every month during the premenstrual phase of the cycle, although there are other factors operative at this time. I'm certain that you have had the experience of gaining six or seven pounds within twenty-four hours of a cocktail party where salty hors d'oeuvres were served. Some overly apprehensive women have noted the simultaneous decrease in the output of urine and because of this, and the leg edema, call frantically on the telephone that they are in heart failure or must have a serious kidney disease. But the human body is a wonderfully balanced machine and within twenty-four hours the excessive water is either excreted, expired, or used in metabolic processes.

Progesterone, made in the ovary, tends to negate the edema-producing effects of estrogen, but some of the newer synthetic progestins do not have this desirable effect and actually potentiate the effects of estrogen. This is particularly true of Enovid, which contains a more estrogenic progestin. But this is an individual problem: some women are just "edema prone." Others, unknown to themselves, ingest fantastically large quantities of salt. Many of my patients tell me they "never add salt" at least at the table, but perhaps they do when cooking, "just a pinch here and a pinch there." For an unpleasant but rewarding surprise, examine carefully a low-salt diet. Look at the condiments and the cooking aids you use. The frequency of "sodium" or sodium chloride may not only surprise you, it may revolutionize your cooking and eating habits.

If you have a problem of weight gain while taking the Pill, your physician may diminish this tendency by selecting a different brand. If the extra weight gain is in the form of body tissue, a pill containing the smallest amount of progestin should be selected. If the weight gain is due to edema, a low estrogen preparation should be used. Norinyl-1, Ortho-Novum-1, Norlestrin, Provest, Ovral and Noriday contain only .05 mg. of estrogen. It has been suggested that the sequential pill causes less edema, but the amount of estrogen they contain does not explain this, for Oracon has .1 mg. and Ortho-Novum SQ, Norquen, and C-Quens .08 mg. In some women it is entirely possible that less fluid would be retained by estrogen alone—even in a little higher dose—than by a combination of a synthetic progestin and a lesser amount of estrogen. Again, it is an individual problem that is solved by trial and error methods alone.

The problem of edema may be relieved by a low-salt diet or a diuretic agent. Diuretics, and there are many, increase the excretion of salt and water and greatly alleviate edema. I usually advise my patients to take a diuretic tablet with breakfast for three or four consecutive days if they feel bloated or notice ankle swelling, then stop for three or four days. If leg cramps or weakness are noted, either the amount of diuretic or length of treatment has been excessive. These symptoms are due to an excessive loss of sodium and potassium and are relieved by taking a small amount of salt and fruit juice high in potassium. A few patients limit the diuretic agent to one or two days each week. Many follow a regimen of Friday and Saturday diuretics and have told me that they feel better and look thinner for the week-end festivities.

In summary, weight gain or weight loss during the use of the Pill depends on five major variables: (1) the nature of the population and their eating habits; (2) the amount of estrogen and progestin in the pill; (3) recent pregnancy or persistent lactation; (4) specific qualities of the progestin, that is, whether it is protein building, protein destroying, or essentially neuter; the ability of the progestin itself to retain salt and water; (5) psychosomatic factors.

IMPROVING THE FIGURE

The breast fetishism that has existed in the United States for many years may cause some readers to believe they can enlarge their bosom by taking estrogen or Enovid. This strikes me as less than an ideal reason to take the Pill, and I do not prescribe it for this indication. Enovid will not cause breast tissue to develop, but it will frequently fill out the tissue already present. Just as in pregnancy, the estrogen and progestin produce water retention and stimulate the growth of glandular tissue and ducts. I have seen many patients increase their bra size after having taken Enovid for several months.

I recall one patient who came to see me in 1958 because of extremely irregular, painful, and excessive menstruation. Both ovaries were enlarged, and at surgery I found extensive endometriosis. After a conservative operation, preserving her uterus and ovaries, I started her on an Enovid pseudopregnancy, giving the Pill *constantly,* not in cycles.

At the time I first examined her, she was an extremely skinny 106 pounds. At the end of six months of constant Enovid, I again examined her and found the pelvic organs to be perfectly normal. A marked improvement in her figure was also apparent. Her weight had increased to 126 pounds, partly because of salt and water retention, but principally because she felt better and ate better. She was most pleased with the increase in the size of her breasts. At her request, I kept her on Enovid for another six months, at the end of which time she moved from Boston to New York and found employment as a showgirl in the Copacabana nightclub. She subsequently began to have normal periods without pain.

I did not see her again for five years, when she returned for a complete physical examination. Her endometriosis remained quiescent and she had no symptoms of any kind. I last heard from her several months ago when she wrote that she had married and given birth to a child. It is hardly routine for women on Enovid to become Copacabana showgirls, but there is no doubt that estrogens and progestins may produce a marked improvement of the under-developed figure—if the basic tissue is present but just under-stimulated.

The Pill has a salutary effect on the figures of some women, but it must be remembered the patient just cited was an unusual situation. The Pill was given constantly and in doses ten to twenty times the usual amount administered today. The search for more potent compounds with increased precision of action has practically eliminated the side effects, both desirable and undesirable.

My advice regarding figure control is, therefore, neither startling or new. An attractive figure depends primarily on your mother and father, your inherited genetic pattern. Starting with your basic given characteristics, you may improve certain aspects of your figure by rigid self-control, diet, and exercise. The most important feature is your desire. If you were fortunate to be given a figure like Venus, your ancestors deserve the plaudits. If, however, you are less well endowed, I suggest that you do not look to the Pill as the answer to your problem.

6. Nausea

The second most common reason for discontinuing the Pill is the side effect of nausea. There is no doubt that estrogen produces nausea or a feeling of queasiness. This is clearly evident in early pregnancy or after oral administration of a synthetic estrogen such as DES (diethylstilbestrol). The exact cause is unknown, but there is no doubt that it is related to the dose and, to a lesser extent, to the type of estrogenic substance administered. The natural estrogen Premarin (sodium estrone sulfate) produces much less nausea than synthetic forms. In some women other gastrointestinal complaints such as cramps or diarrhea may accompany the nausea or appear as independent symptoms.

Nausea occurs most frequently among Pill users giving a history of nausea during pregnancy. Although this gradually disappears by the twelfth week of gestation, a few women note persistence of the symptom. Vomiting may be severe and recurrent with a loss of body fluids. Dehydration ensues, and termination of the pregnancy is occasionally indicated. This disease, known as *hyperemesis gravidarum,* is believed to represent an exaggerated response to estrogen, a response based on psychosomatic factors. Psychiatrists have suggested that hyperemesis represents an unconscious, repressed rejection of the pregnancy with the ejection

68

of stomach contents signifying the body's attempt to empty the uterus. Transferring this reasoning to Pill users, one might speculate that persistent nausea or vomiting represents an underlying guilt feeling and that these symptoms afford the patient a valid reason for stopping the Pill. Certainly the incidence of persistent nausea is minimal in those women who have the greatest motivation for the prevention of pregnancy, for example, in less affluent societies. But hyperemesis of pregnancy is also rare in these individuals.

The nausea induced by oral contraceptives is transient in most women. The incidence is highest during the first month of use, rapidly declines to low levels, and disappears after three or four cycles. I have seen only one or two patients who stated that they were constantly nauseated for one or more years. In the majority of patients nausea is mild and lasts only a few days. Vomiting rarely occurs. However, there are a few women who are unable to tolerate estrogen by mouth, and for them I substitute newer injectable substances. In one of these compounds, Deladroxate, the estrogen is released into the blood very gradually. None reaches the gastrointestinal tract; some of it is undoubtedly metabolized in the liver before reaching areas of the brain where the sensation of nausea is interpreted.

How can nausea be prevented or diminished? First, tell your physician that you are prone to nausea, motion sickness, or have an unstable or easily upset stomach. Mention previous experiences during pregnancy or after taking estrogens. If you have experienced repeated episodes of indigestion, gas, burping, possibly associated with sick headaches, x-rays of the stomach and gall bladder should be done. If these symptoms become aggravated, after starting the Pill, it would be natural to attribute them to estrogen. After your physician has evaluated your history and completed the physical examination, he will, if you are nausea prone, select one of the Pills containing the lowest amount of estrogen.

A second preventive measure was brought to my attention by my nurse. She told me that when she took the Pill (one with .1 mg. of estrogen) before retiring, nausea was excessive. This was prevented completely if she swallowed the Pill with her evening meal.

I frequently give patients an anti-emetic drug to take along with their oral contraceptive, especially during the first cycle or two and if they have informed me of estrogen sensitivity. The dose of anti-emetic is gradually diminished as time goes on.

It is important for the user to understand that nausea, when it does occur, is most often a phenomenon of the first cycle of use. It is unusual for it to continue past the third cycle. Therefore, the best "treatment" for the nausea associated with the Pill is prophylaxis and patience.

7. Breakthrough Bleeding

STAINING," "SPOTTING," or bleeding between menstrual periods ranks third as a reason for discontinuing the Pill. Such complaints are usually referred to as "breakthrough" bleeding because a portion of the endometrium degenerates, that is, it "breaks through" the estrogen stimulation that should keep it intact. By whatever name, the condition is a nuisance to most patients and is disconcerting to others.

The cause of breakthrough bleeding is quite simple. It is due to degeneration of endometrial tissue as a result of inadequate nutrition. During the normal ovarian cycle after bleeding occurs, the estrogen level in the body increases *gradually* up to the time of ovulation. There is a slight drop in the estrogen level at the time of ovulation, but as soon as the corpus luteum is formed, estrogen and progesterone are *gradually* increased for about ten days. I have emphasized *gradually* because it is this aspect of estrogen that prevents bleeding during the normal cycle. Estrogen builds the tissue and blood vessels of the endometrium. Now visualize what happens when the Pill is taken, especially a pill with a low amount of estrogen. The endometrium grows gradually, but if there is an inadequate amount of estrogen to maintain growth, it crumbles. It's something like trying to live on a fixed income when the cost of living increases. Something has to give.

Still another factor must be considered. Remember that I mentioned the extreme potency of the newer progestins and how anti-estrogenic some of them are. This degree of opposition to the effect of estrogen on endometrial growth is sufficient, in many patients, to prevent normal growth of tissue and blood vessels—breakthrough bleeding results.

Two corrective actions may be taken if breakthrough bleeding occurs. These have already been mentioned, but I will repeat them for emphasis. First, double the dose at the first sign of staining. This is particularly recommended if the patient is taking one of the newer brands containing only .05 mg. of estrogen. The doubled dose is continued until the end of the cycle. The usual one-tablet-daily dose is taken in the next cycle. Second, the pill may be stopped and the breakthrough bleeding considered as a regular menstrual period. Pill taking is resumed five days after the onset of flow. Either of these two approaches eliminates the nuisance bleeding for most women.

If breakthrough bleeding persists beyond three or four months, call your physician. It is possible that certain disease processes have developed while you have been using the Pill. I do not imply cause and effect, because these diseases are just as common in nonusers of the Pill. Infections, such as gonorrhea or tuberculosis, may be the cause of persistent bleeding. Or, a small benign tumor, a polyp, may be present. Fibroids cause abnormal bleeding—both in users and nonusers of the Pill. Therefore, don't put your head in the sand and assume the bleeding is pill related. A few simple diagnostic tests will put your mind at rest and proper therapy will put a stop to the bleeding.

If a specific cause for the bleeding cannot be found, I usually prescribe another type of estrogen-progestin combination, varying the amount of estrogen and progestin as the symptoms indicate. In certain patients it may be advantageous to use the sequential pill because of its unopposed estrogen. Don't jump to the unwarranted conclusion that the Pill is not for you on the basis of recurrent breakthrough bleeding of two to three months' duration on one brand. At the same time, when changing from one brand to another, give it and your endometrium a chance. It may take three or four months for compatibility to develop. Most investigators studying the problem of breakthrough bleeding have observed diminished frequency after the first year. Eventually a stable pattern develops and normal or scanty bleeding occurs with clocklike regularity.

The side effects of the Pill still need to be placed in proper perspective. A recent article in *McCall's* magazine by Leslie Aldridge stated,[23] "It's the best contraceptive ever devised. Why then have three million women dropped it?" This article was based on a study of 5,600 pill users, non-pill users, and pill dropouts during the years 1960 through 1965, published in September of 1966 in *Science*.[24] The study was released by the Office of Population Research at Princeton, New Jersey, and was conducted by Professor Charles F. Westoff, Chairman of the Department of Sociology at Princeton University, and Norman B. Ryder, of the Department of Sociology at the University of Wisconsin. Of the total number of 102 dropouts, 20 per cent did so for reasons unrelated to pill side effects. These women desired to become pregnant, reached the menopause, were divorced or separated, or were temporarily estranged from their husband because of war or business. Dropouts were higher during the interval 1960–1965 than at the present because the FDA had imposed a two-year limit on pill usage that was not removed until 1966. The number of women discontinuing the Pill because of this regulation is not stated in the article. Furthermore, the first low-dosage oral contraceptives did not appear until 1964, and since a high proportion of dropouts are due to side effects, it is fair to assume that the rate of dropout due to these effects is presently less than cited in the article.

Of the remaining 80 per cent of women who discontinued the Pill, 15 per cent gave up because of psychological problems. Some just did not like the idea of taking a tablet every day; others worried that it might not be effective; a few thought they might forget to take it. One psychiatrist commented on the insomnia noted by pill users, stating that most patients spent sleepless nights worrying about whether they had or had not taken their pill before retiring.

The remainder of the dropouts, 65 per cent, discontinued the Pill because of unpleasant or frightening side effects, chiefly the weight-gain, fluid-retention, breast-tenderness triad previously mentioned and irregularities of bleeding, mostly of the breakthrough type. With the use of the newer mini-dose preparations I doubt whether the dropout rate will be anything like that reported by Westoff and Ryder. There is always the possibility that some women may even imagine they have certain side effects if they read about them often enough in the newspapers and magazines. Rashes of specific symptoms always appear subsequent to the publication of a new complication. It is interesting to note in the report of Westoff and Ryder that almost 40 per cent of women who *did not* drop out had undesirable side effects that disappeared. Others stated that the side effects persisted but that they were not of sufficient severity to warrant stopping a method of conception control that was 100 per cent effective.

8. The Pill and Your Complexion

No EFFECT of the Pill has received as much publicity as its alleged ability to create a beautiful complexion. The Pill, particularly its estrogen component, has been ballyhooed as being able to prevent and even remove wrinkles and thereby keep a woman's skin "feminine forever." There is both wheat and chaff in these claims, for the Pill may exert both an advantageous and deleterious effect on a woman's complexion. Unfortunately, both the cosmetic industry and some physicians, either through misconception or greed, have enriched themselves by deluding women into believing that an estrogen-progestin pill is a quick route to youth and beauty.

Three basic concepts are important. First, the estrogen in the contraceptive pill has the same hormonal effects as other estrogens given to postmenopausal women to preserve femininity. Second, no additional benefit is gained from rubbing estrogen or progesterone into the skin, over what may be gained from oral administration. Third, it is not necessary to have your own supply of progesterone, nor to take it in a pill to be thoroughly female— unless you consider having a baby to be part of that definition. Progesterone is for pregnancy—nothing more.

To emphasize the latter point, I should say that some of the most beautiful and thoroughly feminine women I have seen are not women at all. They do not menstruate since they have no uterus; they cannot have sexual intercourse since they have no vagina; and, most amazingly, they do not have ovaries. Their gonads are testes situated in the abdomen. This disease, an inherited one, is called "testicular femininization." Now that we understand the endocrine basis, the explanation is easy. Although the testes of these women make a normal amount of male hormone, the organs in their body cannot react to it. Remember earlier I described how estrogen is made from male hormone. The testes of these women also make estrogen and, the way nature arranged things, in order for male external genitalia to develop in the fetus, functioning testes must be present: In the absence of testes as an "organizer," everything "turns out female." So, at the time of puberty, the testes make estrogen. Breast development is excellent, body contour feminine, the skin soft and supple. These individuals look, act, and should be considered as females—but not one drop of progesterone was needed to produce or maintain this feminine appearance, nor will it ever be.

Don't despair for these "girls," however. The gonads are removed because of their tendency to become cancerous; estrogen is given orally *ad infinitum,* and their femininity is retained until the normal process of aging occurs; an artificial but normally functional vagina is constructed. A normal married life is possible —with two exceptions. Since there is no uterus, menstruation and pregnancy are impossible. This "woman" is now comparable to a normal female who has had a hysterectomy and removal of the ovaries.

What does this have to do with your complexion? It should explain that to have a beautiful skin, you need not ovulate, menstruate, get pregnant, or take progesterone. You do need estrogen, health, and the help of heredity.

"BLOTCHINESS" OF THE SKIN

One of the more common and unflattering side effects of the oral contraceptives is a change in skin pigmentation called chloasma or melasma. A significant number of women taking the Pill develop brownish blotches or patches on the skin, particularly on the forehead and cheeks. The discolored areas cannot be distinguished from the "mask of pregnancy," although the latter is usually more deeply colored.

The blotches are not an uncommon side effect. Seventy-two per cent of the physicians surveyed by the American College of Obstetricians and Gynecologists reported having patients with this symptom. The survey indicated that the complaint was more common in the Deep South and along the West Coast than in the less sunny Northeast. One study of 212 patients taking oral contraceptives showed that 29 per cent developed melasma. In my own practice, I see it in less than 5 per cent of the patients, however.

How and why the Pill causes these giant freckles is a puzzle, but it is possible to offer suggestions for prevention and, to a certain extent, palliation.

There is no reason to be alarmed about the blotches. They are not related to skin cancer nor to rashes, allergies, or any other skin disease. They are cosmetically unflattering to some women, but I know others, golfers, tennis players, and swimmers, who find them attractive, perhaps as a badge of their activities.

There are several actions a woman can take to ease the problem. Obviously, face powders or creams can mask the blotches. Another step is to shield the face from the sun as much as possible. A day at the beach accentuates the blotches, since the change in skin pigmentation causes them to darken more than the surrounding areas. When exposed to the sun for any interval, one of the protective creams that filter out ultraviolet rays should be used. These are the rays that produce tanning. One of the screening preparations, Eldopaque, may be used prior to and during exposure to the sun. Redheads with fair skin have found this an excellent method of preventing freckles.

Unfortunately, changing the type or dosage of the Pill does not improve melasma once it has developed. The incidence may be less with the newer mini-dose pills, however. Although the exact cause of freckling is not known, we do know that the deposition of the pigment, melanin, is regulated by pituitary and adrenal function and that melasma is common in pregnancy. In fact, 87 per cent of the patients noting melasma while using oral contraceptives had also noted this condition during pregnancy. Unfortunately, the increased pigmentation tends to remain even after the Pill is discontinued.

In search for a cause, it can be said that melasma does not occur in women taking estrogen alone, nor does it occur when progesterone alone is given. These observations suggest that it is the combination of progestin with estrogen that causes the discoloration. Since all oral contraceptives contain both hormones, including the sequentials, changing the Pill does not ease the condition.

In my experience I've found that most patients accept the blotches as an annoyance and continue the Pill. Their attitude was expressed by one patient who said, "I'd rather be blotchy than pregnant." That seems sensible, if only because pregnancy may cause blotches, too.

ACNE

A significant improvement in acne is one of the major cosmetic effects noted by many users of oral contraceptives. It is known that the male hormone testosterone stimulates the sebaceous glands of the skin to enlarge and secrete sebum. Sebum is an oily material that provides the natural lubrication of the skin. These glands are heavily distributed in facial areas, and over the chest and back. At the time of puberty in the male, the testes increase their secretion of testosterone. In sensitive individuals, the glands are overstimulated, the duct leading from the gland becomes occluded and the liquid sebum solidifies. Skin bacteria invade the area and a small pustule develops. The same process occurs in teenage girls if their ovaries secrete excessive amounts of male hormone.

A time honored treatment in the female has been the use of estrogen alone to suppress the pituitary, rest the ovary, and diminish the secretion of male hormone. During the early 1960's, numerous observations of improved acne were made by patients taking Enovid. The mechanism is identical. However, the original Ortho-Novum, 10 mgs., because it contained an excessive amount of an androgenic progestin, actually produced acne in women who previously had clear skins. Fortunately, the mini-doses of progestin in the newer preparations do not have this effect.

The desire of women for youth and beauty has caused many to look upon the word "wrinkle" as a "dirty word." Personally, I've always felt that the wrinkles that develop as a woman smiles and laughs and registers other emotions give character to her face and add true beauty.

Skin wrinkles are inevitable. They are caused by the tick of the clock. Aging brings wrinkles. An aging woman should accept this as being as inevitable as the sun rising in the east. But how rapidly wrinkles appear in relation to the passage of time depends upon a variety of factors. I have seen women in their thirties, hormonally normal, with many wrinkles, and other women in their fifties with only a few. One reason for this seems to be heredity. At birth a woman has a built-in genetic pattern that predetermines, to a certain degree, the integrity of her skin. This may be modified by health and disease, by obesity, by worry and even by climate. The wrinkling process is slowed if a woman is athletic, eats well, and remains in good health. On the other hand, excessive drying of the skin by wind and sun may predispose to premature wrinkling.

What effect does the estrogen in the Pill—or estrogen alone— have on wrinkles? The supposed therapeutic benefits of estrogen on the skin have been the subject of the aforementioned ballyhoo. It is time, I believe, that some rather positive statements were made about this.

1. Applying estrogen to the skin locally in creams and lotions has no effect—none. The creams may have the effect of cleansing or lubricating the skin and the massage increases the blood supply. But the estrogen does nothing beyond that which a Pill will do, and claims that they do must be considered quackery. After all, from a purely scientific viewpoint, application of an estrogen skin cream introduces three variables: the lubricant, the massage, the hormone. As far as I know, scientific data has not been pub-

lished that proves that topical estrogen alone produces results which are superior to either of the other two methods in the prevention or elimination of skin wrinkles. There is no doubt that a certain amount of estrogen is absorbed through the skin as it is from the vagina. But the absorption rate may be irregular and regulation of the amount of estrogen rubbed in is difficult. One of my patients gave herself so many facial massages with estrogen that her endometrium became excessively thickened and resulted in profuse and irregular bleeding. Her wrinkles, unfortunately, were unchanged.

Wrinkles are caused by sagging or lack of tone in facial muscles, together with changes in the supporting elastic tissue and fat. Obese women are less likely to show wrinkles at an early age, but when they diet and facial fat is lost, they seem to age rapidly.

2. Estrogen, taken orally or by injection, has no effect on wrinkles that already exist. Although estrogen does offer multiple benefits to older women entering the menopause, it does not remove wrinkles. Estrogen cannot turn back the clock insofar as the skin is concerned.

3. It is true, however, that estrogen, administered orally or by injection, *may* diminish the rate at which wrinkles develop. The word *may* is emphasized, because so many other factors must be considered of equal importance. Genetic background, illness or stress may negate any beneficial effects. In my opinion, estrogen may retard the development of wrinkles because the woman feels better, eats better, is more athletic, and has improved protein metabolism. Her mental outlook, if only because she has lost the fear of pregnancy and is enjoying a more loving relationship with her husband, is improved. But let me emphasize one fact, a fact frequently misunderstood by women who have gained their medical knowledge from women's publications. You cannot improve upon the estrogen derived from your own ovaries! What I have suggested as a possible salutary effect of this hormone taken in pill form refers *only* to women who have a demonstrable deficiency of estrogen. In younger individuals, this may be due to congenital absence of ovaries, hysterectomy and ovarian removal, or premature menopause. Women in their thirties and forties who have

normal menstrual cycles with normal flow are not estrogen insufficient and will gain no benefit from any hormonal preparation. If the Pill is desired as an oral contraceptive, that's a valid reason to take it. But don't expect the Pill to do a better job than your own ovary!

So, as far as the skin is concerned, estrogen will not stop the clock or turn it backwards, but it may slow it down for indirect reasons. Therefore, a woman may rightly consider the effect upon the complexion as an advantage of the Pill if she is deficient in estrogen. But she should be mentally prepared for the gracious process of aging. A woman may stay young at heart forever, but I'm afraid her skin must eventually reflect her senior status.

BALDNESS

An infrequent complaint, but one nonetheless heard, is that the Pill causes baldness, which bears the medical terminology of scalp alopecia.

Baldness among women is increasing at a considerable rate. Since six million women are taking the Pill, it is logical to assume that a small per cent of these might develop hair loss for completely unrelated reasons—about the same per cent as in nonusers of the Pill. But when anything unusual happens to a woman taking the Pill, it is the Number 1 suspect.

A possible link between the Pill and baldness was suggested in a report from the Cornell University Medical School. Physicians there described five patients who developed bald spots during or following administration of oral contraceptives. As an isolated report this is not significant, but it is newsworthy. You read it and you worry. A statistician would ask how many women of the same age group, color, and of similar backgrounds were seen with alopecia who were *not* taking the Pill. But even this is not a statistically significant observation. Since the incidence of the complaint is so infrequent, hundreds of thousands of users and nonusers would have to be compared.

There are numerous causes for baldness in women. Tight curlers, nylon brushes, hair straighteners, dyes, and sprays are the most common offenders. Focal areas of baldness may occur after severe infections or high fever. Certain drugs such as heparin, used in treating blood clotting disorders, may result in a loss of hair. Emotional stress, rapid weight loss, malnutrition—even pregnancy itself—all have been implicated in this problem.

The only possible correlation between the Pill and baldness has been the observation of excessive hair loss subsequent to delivery. Dermatologists have long been acquainted with this phenomenon—dismayed women standing before the mirror in tears as their comb dislodges shocks of beautiful hair. But how many baldheaded recent mothers have you seen? The explanation? Excessive hair growth occurs during pregnancy. The excess comes out after delivery and is promptly replaced. For a few weeks, however, areas of the scalp may show through. Time and reassurance cure this problem. It is possible that a similar hormonal rearrangement occurs after discontinuing the Pill, but I must confess that in my twelve years of experience with the oral contraceptives, I have yet to see a patient with extensive alopecia. If the cause were similar to pregnancy, I would expect a higher incidence after cessation of pseudopregnancy, where much larger doses are given on a noncyclic basis. I have seen none in over three hundred patients so treated.

My feeling is that until some specific link between the Pill and baldness is discovered, the condition must be considered coincidental. Baldness is increasing among women because of the reasons noted above. It is unavoidable, therefore, that some women taking the Pill will also develop a similar tendency. If a tendency to excessive hair loss is noted while the Pill is being taken, the advice of a dermatologist should be sought. During the last ten years I have referred no more than six patients to Dr. Walter Lever, Professor of Dermatology at Boston University College of Medicine, and all were referred because of the complaint of "excessive hair loss" shortly after discontinuing the Pill. None of these women had areas of baldness (alopecia) nor did any of them become bald subsequently. Dr. Lever has stated, "There is no known correlation between alopecia totalis (total baldness) or alopecia areata (spotty baldness) and the use of the oral contraceptive agents. This disease is associated with an inflammatory process in the dermis (skin) and is caused by unknown factors but frequently it is of psychosomatic origin." Dr. Lever has commented further that the hair loss following stopping the Pill is a temporary hormonal situation similar to that seen after pregnancy. He has seen no cases of partial or total baldness that he could attribute to the use of the Pill.

9. The Pill and
Your Next Baby

AMONG THE QUESTIONS I am asked most frequently are: If I take the Pill, will I be able to become pregnant when I want to? If I do become pregnant, will the baby be harmed in any way? How soon can I resume taking the Pill after I have a baby?

THE PILL AND FERTILITY

For the woman who has completed her family, subsequent fertility is of no importance. The question of fertility for younger women who plan to use oral contraception for several years is a matter of great importance to both patient and physician. The answer to this question depends, in some measure, on the past obstetrical history of the individual. If pregnancies occurred almost at will prior to pill usage, the chances are excellent that she will conceive quickly after discontinuing them. However, if irregular ovulation or other gynecological diseases such as endometriosis caused a prolonged delay in conception prior to starting the Pill, a similar delay may be expected. Happily, this is not always the case since pregnancy usually brings about improve-

84

ment in endometriosis. Furthermore, this disease is less likely to be aggravated by the scanty menstrual discharge escaping via the tubes into the pelvic cavity that occurs with the newer oral contraceptives. I have frequently noted that pregnancy occurs quite quickly in such patients, occasionally within a month or two.

Many other women may have had a prolonged period of infertility prior to their first pregnancy due to irregular ovulation. The majority of these women usually revert to their prepregnancy status and again find it difficult to become pregnant. A favored few, however, acquire a normal pituitary-ovarian relationship, either because of the pregnancy, the postpregnancy pituitary suppression, or both. In any event, they find themselves pregnant very quickly after stopping the Pill.

Thus, only a minority of women have difficulty in conceiving within a reasonable time. Clinical studies have shown that 75 per cent of women who desire pregnancy conceive within three cycles after stopping the Pill, and 90 per cent are pregnant within one year.

Yet, that minority of women who do not conceive within one year is of concern to physicians. The American College of Obstetricians and Gynecologists survey indicated that 13 per cent of physicians had no patients who had difficulty conceiving after discontinuing the Pill. But 84 per cent said that *some* patients were unable to become pregnant when they wanted to. Almost half the physicians responding to the survey reported this problem occurred rarely. One-third said it happened occasionally.

There are three important facts to keep in mind in considering the effect of the Pill on future pregnancies. First, a woman is not considered infertile unless pregnancy does not occur within one year of regular, frequent intercourse with a male having adequate sperm. Second, 7 per cent of all women are infertile. They will never conceive, and Pill taking has no effect on their infertility. Third, another 3 per cent of women have secondary infertility, that is, after having had one or more pregnancies, they find it impossible to conceive again. It must be assumed that a significant number of women who fail to conceive after stopping the Pill would have been infertile even if they never had taken the Pill.

One of the causes of post-Pill infertility is failure to ovulate. When this occurs, menstruation ceases and a state of *amenorrhea* or "no menstruation" occurs. Again, this may be related to the Pill or it may not. Dr. Ralph Reese of Chicago has commented that one in two hundred or three hundred patients will have a "temporary" amenorrhea after using the Pill, but many of these patients had irregular menstruation even *before* going on the Pill. They have simply reverted to their pre-Pill menstrual pattern.

It is important to realize that the usual causes of ovulation failure may occur in women taking the Pill, as well as in those who are not. During the year or longer of Pill taking, abnormalities in thyroid or adrenal function may occur. Stress factors may affect the hypothalamus and pituitary. Even tumors of various endocrine glands may have developed. It is an error, I believe, to assume that the ovulation failure is *due* to the Pill simply because the Pill was used. In my practice I was able to diagnose tumor of the pituitary gland in two patients referred because of prolonged lack of menstruation after using the Pill. But the diagnosis was possible only because I did a complete survey of the entire endocrine system and x-rays of the skull. If I had considered the amenorrhea to be pill related, the diagnosis would have been missed.

Fortunately, most women who fail to ovulate and menstruate immediately after using the Pill are not doomed to childlessness. In most cases menstruation starts after four to six months. If there are no other causes for infertility, pregnancy usually follows without unusual delay.

If lack of ovulation persists beyond six months, a diagnostic survey is performed. If the survey reveals the only abnormality to be inadequate release of pituitary hormones—and this is the most common abnormality found in these patients—excellent results may be obtained by using one of the newer ovulation-inducing drugs. There are two available, Clomid and Pergonal. Clomid, taken in pill form, stimulates the pituitary to release FSH and LH. Pergonal, given by injection, is derived from the urine of postmenopausal women and *is* FSH, plus a little LH contaminant.*

---

* It so happens that the Cutter Laboratories, Inc., which markets Pergonal, obtains the needed urine from an Italian nunnery. The postmenopausal sisters

These drugs are highly effective, usually producing prompt ovulation. If no other reason for infertility exists, pregnancy usually follows within four or five cycles of treatment.

Nevertheless, the problem of infertility following use of the Pill occurs sufficiently often that many physicians recommend that younger women discontinue the Pill for short intervals periodically. This is particularly important in women who have not demonstrated their ability to become pregnant. My plan is to stop the Pill for three or four months every two years in this age group. The majority will begin to menstruate in four to six weeks and, after two or three normal cycles, the Pill is restarted. Among the physicians surveyed, 44 per cent said they stop the Pill temporarily after four years or less of use. A quarter of the doctors take patients off the Pill for a month or two every two years. As mentioned, I think this is to be recommended particularly for the younger woman who has not been pregnant before.

EFFECTS ON THE NEWBORN

If a woman discontinues the Pill and becomes pregnant, there is not a shred of evidence that her baby will be affected. If the baby is in any way unhealthy or abnormal, the fact that the Pill had been taken previously cannot be correlated with the cause of the misfortune.

After the Pill has been discontinued, its effects do not linger on. Studies of ovaries removed during treatment with oral contraceptives have shown no intrinsic abnormalities in the egg or follicle structure. The ovaries merely rest—as they do during pregnancy. As a matter of fact, in the early 1960's we gave large doses of estrogen-progestin tablets (exactly the same as oral contraceptives) to women who were pregnant and threatening to have a miscarriage. Abnormal babies did not occur more frequently in women who subsequently delivered than in women who had not received the Pill.

---

collected their urine daily and, since a high concentration of FSH and LH are present in the urine of postmenopausal females, the much needed hormones were extracted and crystallized.

Only one special circumstance need be discussed. There would be no point in a woman continuing to take the contraceptive pill while pregnant, but doctors still administer progestins to women with a threatened miscarriage, particularly if the woman has a history of previous miscarriages. The progestin aids both in implantation of the fertilized egg and its subsequent maintenance in the uterus. Physicians select the progestin used for this purpose with care, for it is known that certain androgenic progestins can cause congenital malformations of the external female genital tract in the form of an enlarged clitoris and fusion of the outer lips or vulva. Although these abnormalities are easily corrected surgically, their occurrence is certainly undesirable. These abnormalities occur only in the female fetus (there are no similar effects in the male fetus) when an androgenic progestin is administered *in fairly high doses* during the first four to eight weeks of pregnancy, that is, when these organs are forming. To avoid this complication, physicians choose a progestin that is very similar to that of natural progesterone. Two are presently available, Delalutin and Provera. The latter is the progestin in the oral contraceptive Provest.

In any event, this special circumstance is a problem for the physician. No woman would ever have occasion to take the Pill during pregnancy.

RESUMING THE PILL AFTER PREGNANCY

If a mother is not planning to breast feed her baby, I usually prescribe use of oral contraceptives four to six weeks after delivery. This usually coincides with the first postpartum examination of the patient. Several studies have shown that ovulation occurs about forty to forty-four days following delivery. However, this is not absolute and ovulation may occur sooner. Therefore, it is advisable that other contraceptive methods (condom, diaphragm) be used until effective menstrual cycles have been established.

If the mother is planning to breast feed her baby, some special problems must be considered. It has been accepted therapy for many years to inhibit lactation or secretion of mother's milk by administering large amounts of estrogens or a combination of estro-

gen and androgen. Apparently these hormones are effective because of their ability to inhibit the release of a special hormone,
prolactin, from the pituitary gland. Prolactin stimulates the gland
cells in the breasts to secrete and release milk. The process of
suckling aids in the release of the hormone.

When the Pill was first developed, it was found that higher
dosages of progestin (5 to 10 mgs.) tended to decrease or even
stop lactation. But even when these doses of estrogen and progestin
were present in the Pill, the amount that was excreted in the breast
milk was extremely small. Despite this, a few nursing infants did
develop slight breast enlargement. It must be said, however, that
no specific causal relationship has been established. Some breast
enlargement may occur in infants whose mothers are *not* taking
oral contraceptives. This is due to maternal estrogen that the fetus
absorbed while in the uterus. Dr. Celso Garcia, in his studies in
Puerto Rico, has stated that he has not seen any infant so affected
among the many thousands observed there.[25]

Nevertheless, just to be ultra-safe the pharmaceutical companies
who market the various oral contraceptives advise that the Pill not
be given to nursing mothers. This may be viewed as an example of
the extreme caution with which the Pill is used. There is no evidence that the low-dosage pills now in use (1 and 2 mgs. of progestin) have any effect on lactation at all. Some physicians prescribe
the low-dosage pills to nursing mothers as soon as lactation begins.
Others, more conservative, do not prescribe it at all during the time
a woman is nursing her child. A factor to be considered, since
there is some risk of pregnancy when other means of contraception
are used, is how serious a subsequent pregnancy would be to the
nursing mother. If becoming pregnant would endanger her emotional or physical health, the use of low-dosage pills would seem
warranted. This is most important in many clinics in which a large
percentage of the recently delivered patients are pregnant when
they return six or eight weeks later for a routine checkup—and to
obtain their oral contraceptive prescription.

10. Headaches, "Strokes," and the Pill

THERE IS NO doubt that some women who take oral contraceptives are afflicted with debilitating migraine headaches. A few have been reported to have had fatal vascular accidents called "strokes." But it is also true that women who have never used oral contraceptives have migraine headaches and develop strokes. The question is whether the estrogen and progestin in the Pill in any way cause or aggravate the headaches or strokes. A great deal of research has been and is being done to find an answer.

MIGRAINE HEADACHES

A migraine headache is characterized by an intense, throbbing pain in one side of the head and is usually accompanied by severe nausea. The attack occurs as a result of an artery in or near the brain narrowing and then subsequently expanding. The attacks sometimes last for days and may cause severe discomfort. Since one-third of the physicians surveyed by the American College of Obstetricians and Gynecologists had noted migraine attacks in patients taking oral contraceptives, it seems appropriate to investigate the effects of estrogens and progestins on blood vessels and to determine, if possible, a specific or even nonspecific relationship.

Certain patients report that the Pill causes headaches, and others that their premenstrual headaches disappeared when they used oral contraceptives. Obviously, these must be individual sensitivities to the Pill, just as there are sensitivities to aspirin, penicillin, or sulfa drugs. One woman who had never had headaches before said, "My doctor begged me to try the Pill because I was knocked out every month by menstrual cramps. He was right; I got relief almost immediately from the menstrual pain. But gradually headaches took their place, making me dizzy with pain and nausea. Then one day I went on a trip and forgot to pack the pills. Stopping them cured my headaches the first month."[26]

If that sounds convincing, so does this statement from another patient:

> I have been taking birth control pills for three and a half years under a gynecologist's care and supervision and have been extremely happy with the result. Recently, my physician, who never objected to my taking the pills previously, called and stated that he had read something in the *British Medical Journal* about the combination of birth control pills and migraine headaches resulting in possible stroke. Unfortunately, I suffer from migraine and have for over eight years, four years prior to taking the Pill. My migraine attacks, if anything, have been of less severity since I started taking the Pill. I would also like to add that in addition to the contraceptive action, the Pill has regulated my periods and made my life much simpler, and I have had *no* bad effects from it.

The study to which this patient referred had suggested that oral contraceptives are probably not associated with an increased risk of heart attack but may enhance the chances of a stroke. A more recent study by three neurologists at Western Reserve Medical School in Cleveland had correlated strokelike symptoms with migraine headaches and these in turn with oral contraceptives. The report warned women to stop the Pill promptly if they developed severe migraine, especially if symptoms suggesting an impending stroke, numbness of the extremities or impaired vision occurred simultaneously. This report cited only nine patients and did not claim a statistical relationship between strokes, migraine, and the Pill. The Western Reserve neurologists also stated that electroencephalograms of the nine patients showed exaggerated brain waves —but that these patterns were *not initiated* by the Pill. Stated simply, this implies that certain patients who have a tendency to migraine attacks may have this condition *aggravated,* not caused, by the Pill.

Citing individual patient experience as empirical evidence of cause or aggravation of migraine attacks by oral contraceptives is not acceptable as scientific truth. But these experiences are attractive to news editors and to readers. Contradictory statements by clinical investigators and news agencies only serve to confuse the patient. In my practice, I've seen numerous patients who have typical "menstrual" migraine. These attacks occur just prior to the onset of menstruation when the levels of estrogen and progesterone are low, not high. This suggests that the estrogen and progestin in the Pill do not cause migraine attacks since they substitute approximately normal amounts of each hormone. Furthermore, many women with migraine are appreciably relieved during pregnancy when the estrogen and progesterone levels are extremely high, and I have noted a similar improvement in patients treated with the Pill to effect a pseudopregnancy. Many patients develop migraine attacks during the days when they are not taking the medication. Thus, it would appear that the effects of estrogen and progestin on migraine conditions reflect an individual sensitivity to these hormones and the attack may be precipitated more by *changing* levels of hormones rather than by the Pill itself.

Dr. Eric Nordquist of Lund, Sweden, believes that migraine headaches may be estrogen induced. But evidence to support this theory has not been forthcoming from other clinics. However, the experience of a patient of mine illustrates the point. Following a hysterectomy and removal of both ovaries for a fibroid uterus, I gave this patient various forms of estrogen, both orally and by injection. Each time estrogen was administered, a severe migraine headache developed. However, when a minute dose of estrogen was injected, the migraine attack did not occur. Doubling of the dose immediately induced an attack. Dr. Nordquist has also reported that progesterone and the synthetic progestins *protected against migraine* when they were administered without estrogen in the so-called mini-dose Pill. The dose he gave was too small to prevent ovulation, but pregnancy did not occur because of the progestin's effects on the endometrium and the cervical mucus. In a large number of patients so treated, Dr. Nordquist noted a substantial diminution in the incidence of migraine headaches. Combination estrogen and progestin pills did not offer this protection.

British investigators have recently found that tyramine, an enzyme inhibitor found in foods such as cheese, chocolate, and other dairy products, has been implicated as a precipitating factor in migraine headaches. Large amounts of tyramine, equivalent to the amount in about three ounces of cheese, induced typical migraine headaches in forty of forty-nine patients tested. No evidence is available to suggest that the Pill affects the release or activation of tyramine in the body, but we may soon be reading headlines suggesting that strokes are brought on, in overly sensitive individuals, by a cheese debauch.

If the evidence pro and con concerning the Pill and migraine attacks has seemed confusing, it is an accurate reflection of the present status. We just don't know. The Hellman Committee, in its report to the Food and Drug Administration, stated that more studies were necessary before conclusions about the Pill and migraine headaches could be drawn.

"STROKES"

A migraine headache is debilitating but temporary; a stroke is vastly more serious, may have permanent effects such as paralysis, or prove fatal. Therefore, any evidence that suggests that the Pill is related to the development of strokes gives cause for concern.

Several reports in the medical literature have merely listed the number of patients who sustained strokes while taking oral contraceptives. British physicians reported eight instances between 1962 and 1965.[19] Another report in the United States listed seventeen patients who sustained strokes, four of whom died. In this report, patients had been taking the Pill for one week to three years before the attack occurred. One patient had discontinued the Pill for ten days and another for five months when the stroke took place.

Such studies are not convincing evidence that strokes are *caused* by the Pill. Again, before such a relationship can be proved statistically, it is mandatory that the incidence of the disease be higher in users than nonusers. The above reports list only twenty-five stroke victims in approximately a half-million users. Until recently the incidence of strokes among young, healthy females was thought to be nonexistent or negligible. It was not until comparative studies became necessary that the true incidence became known. In that regard, another British study mentions thirty-nine women between the ages of eighteen and forty-five who had strokes between 1955 and 1965.[27] Of these thirty-nine women, twenty-one had strokes before 1961 when oral contraceptives were first used, and eighteen since then. The study showed that between 1955 and 1960, the number of women in the reproductive age group who had strokes varied from one to five a year. During the post-Pill years of 1961 to 1965, the number varied between two and four cases a year. Not a significant difference!

Any effort to correlate the relationship between stroke and the Pill must necessarily take into consideration the mortality rate in this disease. Vital statistics listing deaths among women from strokes show that they occur from the first year of life through old age. Among white females between the ages of fifteen and twenty-four, the mortality rate from strokes is 1.4 per 100,000 population. Between the ages of twenty-five and thirty-four, the rate increases to 3.4 per 100,000. From thirty-five to forty-four, the rate becomes 10.1 per 100,000. Remember that these figures represent spontaneous occurrence of stroke in all women, *not in Pill users.* By comparison, reports in 1968 by the *British Medical Journal* indicate mortality rates among Pill users from blood clots in the lung and brain to be: 1.5 per 100,000 between twenty and twenty-four years of age and 3.9 per 100,000 for those between thirty-five and forty-four.[11, 12] In other words, prior to age thirty-five, the incidence of death in both situations is about the same, but after that age a woman's chances of dying from stroke increase threefold over that of a woman using the Pill. This does not mean that the Pill protects against death from stroke in women over age thirty-five. In all probability women having previous nonfatal strokes were not placed on the Pill, subsequently died of stroke and the 10.1 per cent per 100,000 incidence is not cluttered by Pill takers.

It is evident that strokes have always occurred among young, apparently normal women. However, since these individuals had not been taking any particular medication, specific causes for the strokes were not sought. For the most part, these deaths were thought to be due to congenital abnormalities in the blood vessels of the brain. They probably still are, and if these unlucky women had been taking aspirin or penicillin, these medications might be indicted as causing the strokes with as much proof as that presented to incriminate the Pill.

To exemplify the relationship of "multiple factors," let me make one further point. Dr. E. Cuyler Hammond, Vice-President of the American Cancer Society's Department of Epidemiology and Statistical Research, has recently made a startling announcement: He found that people who sleep about seven hours a night are less likely to get a stroke or develop heart disease than are those who sleep nine or ten hours. Over the age of fifty, men who sleep nine hours have a death rate from stroke almost twice that of those who sleep only seven hours. Those who sleep as long as ten hours are almost four times as apt to die of stroke. So ladies—if the Pill gives you insomnia—cheer up—it will lessen your chance of dying from stroke!

Nevertheless, manufacturers of oral contraceptives, desiring to be supercautious, warn that the Pill should not be prescribed for the woman who has a history of stroke. Pregnancy is also contraindicated in these patients, but other methods of conception control are advised. Physicians have been warned to discontinue the Pill pending examination of the patient if she complains of sudden partial or complete loss of vision or if there is sudden onset of double vision or migraine headaches. Furthermore, it is suggested that these patients should be examined by an eye specialist. If a peculiar swelling of the optic nerve or a blood-vessel disease is observed, medication should be stopped.

11. The Pill and Liver Disease

About one woman in ten thousand taking the Pill develops a liver dysfunction known as jaundice, which gives a yellowish cast to the skin, nails, and eyes. The rarity of this complication was indicated when only one in twenty physicians surveyed by the American College of Obstetricians and Gynecologists reported encountering it among his patients.

Despite the low incidence of jaundice, the manufacturers of oral contraceptives warn that the medication should not be given to women with a history of liver disease unless tests of liver function indicate a restoration of normal function. Estrogen, progesterone, and the synthetic progestins are "metabolized" in the liver and are converted to compounds that simplify their excretion in the urine and feces. If liver function is inadequate, the systemic effects of each of these hormones may be exaggerated. But this is not the only reason for prohibiting use of the Pill in the presence of liver disease. Of more importance is the fact that certain *progestins* may cause slowing of the flow of bile in the tiny ducts in the liver. If the process is prolonged or excessive, the ducts become plugged with dried bile and the fluid bile backs up into the blood, causing jaundice.

96

It must be emphasized that the Pill does not produce injury to the liver cells. Some investigators have actually obtained small fragments of liver tissue by using an extremely small needle. This procedure, known as "liver biopsy," has provided tissue from hundreds of patients taking the Pill. Microscopic examination has shown the liver cells to be normal and healthy. Several reports from Sweden and Finland indicated that the Pill, if given to pre-menopausal women (age 42 to 52) elevated a specific enzyme in the blood called *transaminase*.[29] Although this enzyme is increased in liver disease, there are many other conditions which do so, also. However, these reports have not been confirmed by other investigators. All reports to date indicate that even though jaundice can develop while the Pill is being taken, liver function quickly returns to normal after it has been discontinued.

Liver function has been thoroughly studied in long-term field trials in Haiti and Puerto Rico.[25] Although the incidence of liver insufficiency is generally higher in these areas than in the United States, jaundice has not been observed among the women studied. The appearance of jaundice is related to the type of progestin used, as well as its dose. For example, the androgenic progestin, norethindrone, was more frequently correlated with jaundice than was norethynodrel (in Enovid) in the early days of oral contraception. But 10 mgs. was the usual dose then as compared to 1 mg. now. I personally observed over one hundred patients who received ten to twenty times the usual dose of Enovid for endometriosis. These patients took six to ten Enovid pills (60–100 mg.) daily, constantly and for periods of time exceeding twelve months. Not one patient developed jaundice in this study.

Recent investigations of patients receiving Enovid have shown a peculiar reduction in the rate of transport of one of the dyes (called BSP) used to measure liver function.[30] In this test a small amount of this dye is injected into an arm vein. The dye goes through the liver and is excreted. The amount of dye retained in the blood after twenty minutes indicates whether liver function is adequate. These studies indicated that the progestin in Enovid interfered with the transfer of the dye from the liver cell into the bile. However, liver biopsies of these patients did not suggest a disease process.

Certain changes noted in the BSP test may represent random variation, since no control groups were studied; that is, the BSP test was not performed on the women before taking the Pill, nor on other nonusers. At the very most, the BSP changes were slight and of no clinical significance since the changes that occurred were reversed as soon as the Pill was discontinued. Furthermore, the same observations of BSP retention have been made in pregnant women. This matter of BSP retention might be summarized by stating that pregnancy, estrogens, and the Pill produce a temporary abnormality that prevents transport of dye across the liver cell into the ducts that drain bile from these cells. All other liver-function tests in this study with norethynodrel remained normal, as did studies of the liver tissue itself.

There is one disease, however, which is a strict contraindication to use of the Pill. The disease is known as "hepatosis of pregnancy" or sometimes as "recurrent jaundice of pregnancy." In this illness, jaundice usually occurs during the latter part of an otherwise normal pregnancy and is usually preceded by an itching of the skin. Some women have had jaundice in three or more successive pregnancies.

The precise cause of pregnancy hepatosis is not known, but there seems to be an inherited tendency toward its development. Furthermore, the disease has a geographic pattern, since many patients have been reported in the Netherlands and South America. It is a rare disease, one investigator reporting only 11 patients with jaundice among 38,000 pregnancies, an incidence of 1 in 3,489. In any event, a history of severe or generalized itching during pregnancy or its occurrence while taking the Pill should be regarded as an early sign of possible impending jaundice and use of oral contraceptives should be terminated.

12. The Pill and Diabetes

Diabetes (correctly *diabetes mellitus*) is a disease of metabolism but really should be considered an endocrine disorder. It occurs as a result of an insufficiency of insulin—a hormone made in special cells of the pancreas. Diabetes is an inherited disease in which the body cannot make full use of some of the foods we eat, mainly the carbohydrates or sugars and starches. The pancreas, a large gland lying beneath the stomach, cannot make enough insulin available to burn the foods as energy or store them in the liver for future use. The starches and sugars build up in the blood but eventually pass through the kidneys and into the urine. The kidneys extract large quantities of water from the blood to excrete the excess sugar. So, one of the symptoms of diabetes is frequency of urination with passage of large quantities of urine. This water must be replaced, so another symptom is that of extreme thirst. The loss of carbohydrate energy in the urine is responsible for another symptom, hunger. Despite the excessive caloric intake, weight loss, even emaciation, may occur.

It is estimated that there are more than 2,750,000 known diabetics in the United States. In addition, there are about 1,250,000 people who are unaware of having diabetes, and more than 3.5 per cent of the total population are presently destined to become diabetic. It occurs with much greater frequency among women than men.

There is no evidence that oral contraceptives *produce* diabetes, but investigators are concerned about a specific effect of the Pill that may expose a latent tendency to develop the disease. In one study, one user in every four utilized blood sugar at a slower rate than normal.

It has been known for quite some time that the blood-sugar levels are elevated in some women during pregnancy. Such women may also show sugar in the urine, but after the pregnancy has been terminated, both the blood and urine tests return to normal. A certain percentage of these women will develop true diabetes some years after pregnancy.

Thus, an important question to be answered is whether the Pill, if used for prolonged periods, is likely to convert latent diabetes into the active disease. Considerable research on this relationship has already been accomplished, but ironclad conclusions are not available. One of the leaders in this field, Dr. William Spellacy, has speculated that "There is a possibility that some may have developed permanent changes in their sugar metabolism, but we don't know yet whether they will go on to develop true diabetes."[31]

The Hellman Committee, in its report on the safety of oral contraceptives to the Food and Drug Administration, stated that data on the effects of the Pill on sugar metabolism in experimental animals and in women are contradictory. The committee noted that abnormal glucose (sugar) tolerance tests have been observed in as many as 40 per cent of women taking the Pill. Among women with a family history of diabetes, the abnormal tests were even more frequent. It was also noted that insulin levels were above normal in "supposedly normal" women taking oral contraceptives. This is understandable, since more insulin would be needed to burn the excessive sugar in the blood. In addition, it is known that some diabetic women require larger injections of insulin while taking the Pill. The Hellman Committee reported, however, that all of these changes regress after the Pill has been discontinued and are similar to those observed during a normal pregnancy. It is not known whether pregnancy can cause diabetes, although diabetes is more prevalent among women having had several pregnancies.

The relationship between oral contraceptives and abnormal glucose tolerance tests may be less a cause for concern than previous reports have indicated Dr. Paul Beck and his co-workers at the University of Colorado concluded that the Pill appeared to be significantly less likely to cause diabetes than normal pregnancy. They studied twenty-seven women with a family history of diabetes during the latter months of pregnancy and found all glucose tolerance tests to be abnormal. After delivery, all women began oral contraceptives and two weeks later they were retested. Abnormal glucose tolerance was found in only three patients, and these were in a group of twelve classified as having "pregnancy diabetes" when previously tested. After two weeks to six months on the Pill, no additional women showed abnormal glucose tolerance.

Dr. Beck suggested that the oral contraceptives alter the glucose tolerance test in a way quite different from that seen in pregnancy or induced by the administration of cortisone-like hormones. Whereas the latter are due to inhibition or retardation of insulin secretion by the pancreas, the oral contraceptives increase the resistance of tissues to insulin so that it cannot function normally to lower blood sugar. Dr. Beck also felt that the oral contraceptives might unmask diabetes in some, but not all, individuals with undetected disease. Pregnancy, or the administration of cortisone, will do a much better job of unmasking these patients, he concluded.

Dr. Jerome Conn of the University of Michigan, an outstanding researcher in this field, commented, "The question of *possible* adverse effect of oral contraceptive agents on carbohydrate tolerance and the development of diabetes must be kept in proper perspective." It has been shown that a diabetic glucose tolerance curve may be produced in *essentially anyone* with a large enough dose of corticosteroids. A corollary might be that a diabetic glucose tolerance curve might also be produced in *essentially anyone* if a large enough dose of estrogen-progestin compound is administered. But doses are going down—not up. This is a far cry from the statement published in the *Lancet* in 1967 that "It may be wise to avoid these drugs [the Pill] in women with known abnormalities of glucose tolerance and possibly also those with a family history of diabetes." According to the work of Dr. Beck, pregnancy should also be avoided by patients in this category, but I seriously doubt if many obstetricians will follow this advice.

I can summarize the relationship between diabetes and the Pill in one short sentence: There is no reason for you to worry about the Pill making you a diabetic any more than pregnancy doing the same thing. However, physicians are cautious about prescribing the Pill for potentially diabetic women; but who is a latent diabetic? One reliable tip is a history of having delivered unusually large babies of nine pounds and over. A family history of diabetes or recurrent fungus infections of the vagina will alert the physicians to obtain blood sugar tests, since tests of the urine are not sufficiently precise.

The majority of specialists in obstetrics and gynecology prescribe the Pill for women who are already diabetic. Three-quarters of the physicans polled by the American College of Obstetricians and Gynecologists reported that they give the Pill to diabetic patients. When this is done, the patient should be observed more frequently by the physicians managing her diabetes. Increase in the level of blood sugar may necessitate changes of insulin dosage or rearrangement of diet, or both. There is no doubt, however, that the risks associated with use of the Pill do not even approach those due to pregnancy.

The work of Dr. Priscilla White at the Joslin Clinic in Boston is of interest in regard to the effect of hormones and pregnancy on diabetes. For many years, Dr. White has treated all pregnant diabetic patients with extremely large doses of estrogen and progesterone. Dr. White observed that the use of these hormones materially diminished the high fetal mortality rate usually found in diabetic patients. Since Dr. White's patients were classified as "severe" or "very severe" diabetics, her results are all the more remarkable. A few obstetricians have disagreed with Dr. White, feeling that the improved fetal mortality rate was due more to her personal attention and diabetic management than to the hormones.

Despite the objection, it is obvious that the tremendous doses of the hormones did not adversely affect the state of the diabetes.

Dr. John Rock has commented on the relationship of the Pill to diabetes in a very practical way. He said it might be a good thing to know if the patient is prediabetic before she becomes pregnant. If the oral contraceptives permit early diagnosis of this condition, one could then caution her about the number of pregnancies she could safely have in the future.

13. Miscellaneous Complaints and Complications

As a result of the estrogen in the Pill, certain minor complaints and three rather serious complications have been reported. The complaints are those of vaginal discharge and swelling of various parts of the body. The latter is known to physicians as edema and represents a tendency to retain salt and water. The complications are those of enlargement of benign tumors of the uterus, known as fibroids, premature suppression of growth, and eye abnormalities. The complaints may be avoided by selection of the proper estrogen-progestin combination together with a low-salt diet and a medication that increases the excretion of salt and water. The complications may be avoided by a careful pelvic examination, proper selection of the patient for treatment, and judicious consultation when unusual symptoms occur.

VAGINAL DISCHARGE

An occasional complaint may be noted by a particularly fastidious woman that a sticky, mucoid, white discharge has occurred subsequent to use of the Pill. This is really a normal, almost physiological reaction of the glands that line the inner portion of the cervix to the estrogen component of the Pill. The same situation exists in the adolescent female when the ovaries begin to secrete estrogen. In some girls it persists into adult life, and in others it is minimal or occurs just at the time of ovulation.

Normally the vagina is moist, occasionally to the extent that a discharge stains the underclothing. This normal moisture consists of a mucoid substance from the glands of the cervix and the exudation from the vaginal walls. The color is white and there is no odor. The term leukorrhea has been given to this discharge (Greek: *leukos*—"white," plus *rheein*—"to flow"), and a minimal amount is normal in all females with adequate ovarian function.

If discharge is more than minimal, it is probably due to abnormal conditions such as an infection or ulceration (sometimes called an erosion) of the cervix or one of the several different types of vaginal infections. In the latter case, the discharge is rather profuse and usually causes itching, burning, and inflammation of the vulval skin.

Three of the most common types of vaginal infections are the yeast infections (known as monilia), trichomonas infestations, or an acute infection of the vaginal lining due to certain bacteria. These are not venereal diseases, but each is capable of producing discharge with itching and burning. Occasionally two, and rarely three types of organisms are present at the same time. The diagnosis is made by examination of the discharge under the microscope or by specific cultures in a laboratory.

Trichomonas and bacterial infections are not seen more frequently in women using the Pill, but yeast infections are becoming a more frequent problem. This is probably due to specific changes in the lining cells of the vagina that permit the growth of yeasts and fungi. Apparently the combination of estrogen and progestin increases the concentration of certain carbohydrates in the vaginal cells, thus creating an ideal milieu for growth of these organisms.

Yeast infections are rather common during pregnancy, in the elderly, in association with diabetes, and following the use of antibiotics such as penicillin or tetracycline. In many pregnant patients the problem is controlled by the recurrent use of Mycostatin suppositories or vaginal creams such as Sporostacin or Candeptin. However, some patients develop a resistance even to these medications, and the old-fashioned remedy, painting the vagina with gentian violet, frequently is necessary. As you might expect, the yeast infection in a pregnant, diabetic patient is extremely difficult to manage.

If a yeast infection occurs in a patient taking the oral contraceptive, several methods of therapy are available. First of all, overt diabetes or a tendency toward the development of this disease should be excluded. This is done with a blood test. Second, if the patient is taking an antibiotic, I recommend use of an anti-fungal suppository or cream during the entire time the antibiotic is being administered. Apparently the combination estrogen-progestin oral contraceptives are more inclined to produce fungal infections than the sequential pills. Thus, substitution of one of these agents may be beneficial. Some patients, however, seem to be predisposed to fungal infections even while using the sequential Pill. Some degree of protection is afforded if the patient uses the suppositories or cream during the last five days of the Pill cycle and then again for four or five days after the menstrual period. This becomes rather tedious for many patients, and they may elect to discontinue the Pill. In a few individuals, I have used the newer "mini-progestin" pill, since it contains no estrogen and the progestin itself is actively anti-estrogenic. Another method employs injections of Depo-Provera, a potent progestin, at monthly or trimonthly intervals. While the latter two methods are effective in the control of fungus vaginitis, they have not yet been approved by the FDA for contraceptive use. I have seen no pregnancies in patients receiving Depo-Provera, but the use of mini-dose progestins has not afforded complete protection. I have no doubt that these methods will eventually be made available to the public.

Trichomonas vaginitis occurs in women taking the Pill, but its incidence is not increased beyond that seen in nonusers. The discharge is quite easily recognized, being white or greenish tinged, foamy, and having a characteristic fetid odor. By comparison, the discharge of fungus origin is thick, almost like cream cheese. It is odorless, and occasionally thick white plaques adhere to the vagina or vulva. Trichomonas is readily cured by administration of an oral medication, Flagyl, but it is necessary for the husband and wife to take the tablet for ten days. There is no contraindication for the use of Flagyl in women taking the Pill, and the only side effect is occasional nausea or a "brassy" taste in the mouth.

In addition to the vaginal discharges from fungi and trichomonas, women using the Pill may develop an acute bacterial infection. The most frequent offenders are bacteria from the intestinal tract. These may reach the vagina via soiled sanitary napkins or by improper douching methods. Occasionally the bacteria are introduced at the time of intercourse, particularly if the vaginal lining is abraded or torn. Every so often I see a patient with a foul-smelling, purulent discharge. The diagnosis is obvious as the patient enters the examining room—only a "lost" and degenerated vaginal tampon causes an odor of such intensity. The bacterial causes of vaginitis usually respond rapidly to treatment if a culture is taken, the organism identified, and specific treatment begun.

Another discharge noted frequently in women using oral contraceptives is caused by an ulceration (sometimes called an erosion) of the cervix. As stated earlier in this chapter, estrogen stimulates growth of the glands that line the inner and upper cervix. The function of these glands is to provide a clear mucus for the transport of sperm at the time of ovulation. In pregnant patients, and in users of oral contraceptives, these glands are excessively stimulated by estrogen and progesterone (or progestin). Eventually the glandular portion of the cervix literally overflows onto the portion of the cervix that protrudes into the vagina. When the physician examines the cervix, he sees this red, velvety, glandular portion overriding the normal tissue. Although misnamed an erosion, the condition is really an *eversion*. Treatment is quite simple. Pap smears or biopsies are taken to prove the identity of the process. Then the eversion is cauterized by an electric instrument, an office procedure. This eliminates the abnormally placed glandular tissue, and the cervix quickly covers itself with normal cells.

It is important to distinguish between the various types of vaginal infections that cause discharge in order to institute effective treatment. This obviously requires the diagnostic skills of a physician. Do not assume that the discharge you have now is the same as the one you had a year ago. Furthermore, don't treat yourself with an outdated cream or suppository. In a year's time, a very early cancer *in situ* of the cervix might have developed. I insist, therefore, that all my patients with unusual or excessive discharge have a pelvic examination, visualization of the cervix and vagina, Pap smear, and examination of the discharge under the microscope. In certain instances, biopsies of the cervix and bacteriological cultures are indicated to make a precise diagnosis. Remember also that any bloody or blood-stained discharge, apart from menstruation, calls for immediate investigation by a physician.

FLUID RETENTION (EDEMA)

Despite the numerous advantages of estrogen cited by biologists and physiologists, it is not an ideal hormone for the human female. If I were to redesign it, there are many properties that might well be eliminated. Not the least of these is the propensity of this substance to retain fluid in almost all tissues of the body. Women describe the effect quite realistically. They feel bloated, waterlogged, or, as one patient told me, "like a sponge left in the bathtub overnight."

The fluid retention due to estrogen is quite a simple problem. It is due to an increased reabsorption of sodium chloride (salt) and water by the kidney. Instead of being excreted in the urine, the water and salt recirculate in the blood and are deposited in the tissues. As the tissues swell, a myriad of symptoms appear: puffiness of the feet and ankles, skin itching, headache, dizziness, blurring of vision, lethargy, weight gain, and increased breast tenderness. Occasionally salt and water retention elevate the blood pressure.

The symptoms of fluid retention may be greatly alleviated if the physician selects an oral contraceptive with the lowest amount (.05 mg.) of estrogen. Further relief is afforded by the intermittent use of diuretics to increase excretion of salt and water from the kidneys. In addition, the patient should be cautioned against the ingestion of salt in any form, and she should avoid canned foods with preservatives containing sodium. In certain patients, the body eventually accommodates to the "estrogen load" and the fluid retention is dissipated. In others, a peculiar tendency to edema persists and constant vigilance is necessary.

GROWTH SUPPRESSION

The effects of estrogen on linear growth have been known for many years, but only recently have these effects attracted the attention of physiologists and endocrinologists. As a matter of fact, the problems of human growth have received scant attention despite their importance. Only 4 per cent of women in 1900 were over 5 feet 7 inches tall, compared to 20 per cent today. By virtue of modern pediatric care, avoidance of childhood diseases, improved hygiene and nutrition, there is evolving a much taller American woman. Excessive height in some girls is a social handicap, and for some it may prove to be an economic drawback. The opposite problem, deficient stature, may be of equal or greater importance.

The evidence that estrogens are capable of arresting growth is available in nature's own experiments. In disorders of the adrenal gland or ovaries in which an excess of estrogen is secreted, an early acceleration of growth is followed by premature fusion of the epiphyses (the growing ends of the long bones) and consequent decrease in stature. This observation has led endocrinologists to administer estrogens as growth inhibitors to girls whose ovaries are exceptionally slow to mature and who might reach excessive height.

Because of this property of estrogen, the brochure that accompanies all oral contraceptives states, "Because of the effects of estrogens on epiphyseal closure, this preparation should be used judiciously in young patients in whom bone growth is not complete." But this is nothing new, and this admonition is simply a reiteration of a precept of good medical practice. From a practical standpoint, however, the indication for the use of oral contraceptives in girls who have not as yet begun to ovulate and menstruate is rare indeed. I cannot remember ever having had such a patient, except possibly one with a rare absence of the ovaries (Turner's Syndrone). In patients with this disease we use the estrogen-progestin sequential agents to provide needed hormonal support and to develop the breasts and genitalia, not as a contraceptive since these patients are sterile. But a physician would never think of initiating this treatment until the patient had attained her full height.

Once the process of ovulation and menstruation has been established, the amounts of estrogen made by the ovaries far exceed that administered in the Pill. Thus, the epiphyses will already have been acted on by the patient's own hormones and subsequent use of oral contraceptive agents would be of no significance.

EYE COMPLICATIONS

Probably the most cruel and unfair allegation made against the Pill is that it causes blindness. If one wished to create the maximum fright in users of the Pill, this certainly would accomplish the purpose. As far as I know, there is absolutely no basis for such a cause-and-effect relationship. Of course individual case reports may cite blindness occurring in users of oral contraceptives, but blindness may occur in women taking aspirin, cortisone, or penicillin.

There is no doubt that various symptoms such as double or blurred vision, excessive tearing, or "spots" in the visual field do occur. A cautious gynecologist will refer such a patient to an eye specialist, since any intercurrent eye disease may have developed while the Pill was being taken. One prominent New York City ophthalmologist has commented, "I have patients with these complaints every few weeks. Usually I find no pathology. The symptoms seem to be caused by muscle fatigue which I attribute to worry over the Pill."[26]

On the other hand, certain experts believe the Pill may affect the blood vessels of the eye; reports of blood clotting in the central vein behind the eye have appeared in the literature. Conclusions regarding the effect of the Pill could not be made since these individuals had not had ophthalmoscopic examinations prior to their accident. In Chapter 1, a study by Dr. Elizabeth Connell of New York Medical College was cited.[10] She found that 80 per cent of 389 women had eye abnormalities *before using the Pill.* Most of these were not serious from the standpoint of visual damage, but if they had been observed after the Pill had been started, a good many erroneous conclusions might have been drawn.

In 1965, an article in *Good Housekeeping* cited a report that patients taking oral contraceptives had developed papilledema, a serious condition affecting the major nerve to the eye. The authors of the report made no comment about the Pill *causing* the disease, they simply wished to note the simultaneous occurrence of the two. A report in the *British Medical Journal* in 1967 described two patients who developed partial blindness "shortly after" starting oral contraceptives. Both of these patients had a previous history of migraine, and the blindness followed another attack. This type of blindness is a rare aftermath of migraine headache, but it is well known to neurologists. The "natural" inclination is to state that the Pill caused the migraine attack—and the migraine attack caused the blindness. Again this is after-the-fact reasoning. It is difficult to rationalize, physiologically, that the small amounts of estrogen and progestin in the Pill incited the attack since, if the pills had been taken for only a few days, the patient's own estrogen level would have exceeded that in the Pill. One might speculate that these patients were sensitive to the progestin, but one might also suggest that the migraine attack was brought on by worry that the Pill might have some deadly effect. In any event, as a result of these reports, the brochures accompanying the Pill include a warning against continued use if visual defects occur. Again, this is good standard medical practice. I might add that during my twelve years of experience with estrogen-progestin compounds, I have not seen one patient develop any serious eye complication.

FIBROID TUMORS

One of the complications associated with the Pill is their effect on the growth rate of fibroid tumors of the uterus. These are benign growths that usually are symptomless and shrink during menopause. But when fibroids grow rapidly, they distort the lining of the uterus, resulting in abnormal bleeding. Occasionally a hysterectomy is necessary to control excessive bleeding, but in young patients the fibroids may be removed, preserving the uterus and thus subsequent pregnancies. I have removed as many as seventy-five small fibroids and reconstructed a normal-appearing uterus in an effort to preserve fertility.

There is no evidence that the Pill causes fibroids, but more than half the specialists surveyed are convinced the Pill increases their rate of growth and my experience has been similar. This enlargement is usually reversible if the Pill is discontinued.

Gynecologists have known for a long time that estrogen, if given in large enough amounts for a prolonged period of time, will stimulate the growth rate of fibroids. Therefore, it is the estrogen in the Pill, not the progestin, which complicates treatment with oral contraceptives. In my practice, if a patient has a small fibroid and desires to take the Pill, I select a brand with the lowest content of estrogen and the highest amount of an anti-estrogenic progestin. There are now half-a-dozen brands available which contain only .05 mg. of estrogen. I then insist the patient be examined every three months. If intermittent or excessive bleeding occurs, or if the fibroid enlarges, another method of contraception is substituted. At the present time, I am using Depo-Provera injections in such patients, since this compound is not estrogenic. One of the newer mini-progestin pills (without estrogen) might be utilized or a diaphragm might be suggested. Intrauterine devices are contraindicated in the presence of fibroids.

14. The Pill and Cancer

Few words in the English language create so much fear as the descriptive term *cancer*. Cancer is not a specific disease. Used in the broadest sense, it includes a multitude of diseases which have one thing in common—they are *malignant*. This implies that cell growth has lost its orderly pattern and has been replaced by rapidly growing, lawless cells that respect no boundaries. It is this aspect of cancer that eventually causes death, the ability of these cells to spread to other areas of the body, to vital organs such as the brain or liver, that differentiates a *malignant* tumor or growth from a *benign* one. But all cancers are not identical, either in appearance or in their potential to spread, or, as physicians say, to metastasize. The usual type of skin cancer remains localized and does not spread into adjacent tissue until very late in its development. But another type of skin cancer, melanoma, spreads its cells rapidly by invading the blood stream. The former cancer is, therefore, almost a benign form, whereas the latter is frequently lethal.

In recent years considerable progress has been made in treating cancer with drugs and radiation therapy. Despite these advances, the word cancer still connotes pain, a long and expensive illness, radical surgery, and death. Therefore, any relationship between a specific medication and this disease is viewed with suspicion and alarm.

Since its discovery, many women and a few physicians have expressed vague, unspecified fears that the Pill might, over a long period of time, initiate the development of cancer of the breast or endometrium. This fear is a strange phenomenon, for it persists despite lack of confirmatory evidence of cause and effect and despite contrary evidence that the Pill has been shown to prevent the development of *premalignant* phases of endometrial cancer.[2]

Apprehension that the Pill causes cancer is not shared by the majority of physicians. Reporting on seven years of experience with the Pill, 99 per cent of specialists surveyed by the American College of Obstetricians and Gynecologists stated that they did not correlate breast or endometrial cancer with use of the Pill. The specialists' virtually unanimous statement agrees with the reports of several research studies, particularly data gathered in Puerto Rico where women have taken the Pill for twelve years.

There is one aspect of the problem, however, that remains unanswered. This concerns the time lag or latent period between exposure to agents that cause cancer and the actual development of the disease. The Hellman Committee, in its report to the Food and Drug Administration, said, "It is known that all human carcinogens [an agent causing cancer] require a latent period of approximately one decade before exerting their result. Hence any valid conclusion must await accurate data on a much larger group of women studied for at least 10 years." This conclusion is based on accepted data which indicate that cancer does not develop overnight. Many forms of cancer are preceded by a preliminary stage of the disease known as "cancer *in situ*." During this phase, normal cells become precancerous. But not every cancer *in situ* becomes malignant. In the case of the cervix, the vast majority would probably do so unless some form of treatment is initiated. The period of development of cancer of the cervix from cancer *in situ* approximates seven to ten years. It is for this reason that the Hellman Committee reserved judgment on this most important correlation. Observations on the first group of patients treated ten years ago are now being collected and analyzed. But the sample is small. The next five years should provide sufficient patients from which conclusive data may be derived. Meanwhile, there is no statistically valid basis for linking the Pill to the various cancers that occur in the female.

CANCER OF THE BREAST

Ovarian estrogen and progesterone have a specific effect upon a woman's breasts. Similarly, synthetic estrogen and progestin stimulate breast tissue. The effects of certain brands of pills on breast size have already been discussed. In addition, some women complain of breast soreness or tenderness when they begin to take the Pill. This is the result of temporary engorgement of breast tissue. This discomfort usually diminishes in succeeding cycles, however. Occasionally a small amount of secretion may be noted, but this occurs more frequently after cessation of a "pseudopregnancy" for endometriosis. Only rarely is nipple secretion observed following use of the Pill for contraception. There is no connection between these temporary side effects and breast cancer. Persistent breast secretion may occur in patients with pituitary tumors, and a bloody discharge is usually due to a benign growth, a papilloma, in one of the breast ducts. Neither is pill correlated.

In the twelve years I have been prescribing the Pill, I have seen only one patient develop breast cancer. Perhaps the age group is too young to draw valid conclusions. Yet I see numerous patients in their forties with breast cancer who have been taking no medication whatsoever. Remember that breast cancer affects one of every sixteen women—pill or no pill. Remember, also, that the incidence of this disease has not changed during the last thirty years —three decades during which all varieties of estrogenic substances have been administered. The Hellman Committee reported only one patient among the millions of Pill users who developed breast cancer. The committee concluded: "If the oral contraceptives are at all carcinogenic for the human breast, they cannot be very potent and the occurrence from this cause must be extremely rare." I am in accord with this conclusion.

Nevertheless, the FDA, in its desire to be super-cautious about the Pill, has stated that "The relationship of the oral contraceptives to breast cancer in the human being is unknown." This interpretation is valid, but it encourages an unspecified fear that the Pill *could* cause breast cancer. A similarly valid conclusion might be made in regard to the use of estrogens given for prolonged periods of time for painful menstruation, irregular bleeding, endometriosis, menopause, after hysterectomy and removal of the ovaries, or in women born without ovaries. Certainly these women, particularly the latter two groups, will take estrogens for a much longer period of time than will women using oral contraceptives. But I have never seen a warning by the FDA or by a pharmaceutical company that stated that "The relationship of estrogens to breast cancer in the human being is unknown." Logically, there is no reason to make such a statement, since the incidence of breast cancer in women who have taken estrogens for twenty or thirty years is *not* higher than in women who have not used this hormone.[32] In the 1967 edition of *New Drugs Evaluated by the A.M.A. Council on Drugs*,[33] the statement appears that in more than 30 years of increasing use of estrogens, accumulated statistics have not shown any significant change in the incidence of breast or uterine cancer. Why, then, would the addition of a synthetic progestin to estrogen cause investigators to think that this *combination* might cause breast cancer?

The basis for apprehension is experiments using the mouse and the dog. Investigations in mice indicated that breast cancer could be produced if large doses of estrogen were given for prolonged periods of time. But none of these animals received a progestin at the same time the estrogen was given, and progestins are known to have an anti-estrogenic effect on many tissues. Among sex hormones, estrogens exert an effect particularly on the tissues of the vagina, endometrium, and mammary gland. Yet they are by no means *carcinogens*. They do not have the typical chemical constitution of carcinogens and, furthermore, enormously high doses were necessary to produce cancer of the mammary gland in the particular strain of mice tested. Actually, the tumor rate was not increased; merely the time at which the tumors became manifest was accelerated. In the mice, the incidence of spontaneous cancer was so high that if allowed to live their natural lifetimes, more than 50 per cent would have developed mammary cancer. As for dosage, the susceptible mouse was given half its body weight for one-fourth of its life span. It has been suggested that the "cancerogenic" effect of estrogen is due to the fact that this hormone causes an increased number of cell divisions. The affected cells are thus more susceptible to *existing* cancer-producing stimuli, which may be present at all times in certain individuals. Furthermore, there is good evidence to suggest that the effect of the progestin is to negate the active growth of cells brought about by estrogen.

Another bit of hormonal evidence is available regarding breast cancer. It has been known for some time that breast cancer is less prevalent among women who have had many pregnancies and nursed their babies. This diminished incidence could be related to the process of nursing, but it might also be related to the high estrogen and progesterone levels that occur during pregnancy. Reasoning from a purely practical standpoint, it might be concluded that the breast was designed for the production of milk and that the interruption of cyclic estrogen-progesterone stimulation acts to prevent the development of cancer. The spinster has neither of these benefits. Her breasts are stimulated month after month by fluctuating levels of estrogen and progesterone. The hyperhormonal state of pregnancy never occurs. The formation of milk is denied. The only valid reason that is acceptable to me correlating the Pill and breast cancer is that of pregnancy prevention and the absence of lactation. But the Pill should be used for *spacing* conception, not for its permanent prevention.

Despite the lack of definitive evidence linking the Pill to breast cancer, fear persists. The most recent manifestation of this uncertainty is the furor regarding use of the Pill by women who have a pronounced family history of breast cancer.

There is no doubt that there is an inherited tendency for some women to develop this malignancy. A woman's chance of breast cancer increases twenty-eight times if her mother had this disease and sisters have an increased risk forty times as great as other women. But the Hellman Committee gave no indication that the use of the Pill would increase the possibility of *any* women developing a breast malignancy—whether or not a family history of this disease was present. Furthermore, the authors of the most recent paper on this subject, published in the *New England Journal of Medicine,* concluded, "The facts merely indicate that oral contraceptives have an impact on breast physiology and anatomy. They do *not* establish any clear association with breast cancer itself." It seems illogical to me, therefore, to single out these individuals, simply on the basis of their family history, as a group who should not receive the Pill. Certainly the most important aspect regarding mammary carcinoma is its prevention. At present, the only effective method is early diagnosis by palpation or x-ray.

For the past eight years I have given oral contraceptives to patients whose family history included mammary carcinoma in mothers or sisters. However, I inform these patients of their increased cancer potential and I insist on a thorough examination of the breasts at intervals of three to six months. Removal of any lump is mandatory, and mammograms (soft tissue x-rays of the breasts) are done whenever a suspicion of a mass arises. During these eight years, I have seen only one patient who developed breast cancer while using oral contraceptives. In this patient, I was able to detect a pea-sized mass at the time of her regular examination. I immediately performed a radical mastectomy and was pleased to note that the cancer was localized to the area of the mass; all lymph nodes in the armpits were free of tumor. Her prognosis is excellent, an 80 per cent chance of a five-year survival. But I wonder if her cancer would have been detected at this early stage if she had not been obliged to have regular examinations.

There is no doubt that a statistical problem exists, however. With a four-year follow-up of women age twenty to thirty, a sample of 20,000 women taking the Pill would be required to have a reasonable chance of detecting a twofold increase in the incidence of breast cancer. The answer should be forthcoming in the near future.

The administration of estrogen to women in the childbearing period of life or at the time of menopause may aggravate *already existing* breast cancer. It is obvious, therefore, that the Pill is contraindicated in such patients. There is no doubt that breast cancer is frequently a hormone-dependent tumor. For example, women who have had their ovaries removed early in life seem less likely to develop breast cancer. Similarly, if breast cancer has spread throughout the body, removal of the ovaries will frequently produce dramatic, although temporary, improvement. This is undoubtedly due to the removal of most of the body's estrogen. As further proof, a secondary improvement may be secured even after further spread of the disease by removing the adrenal glands, the only other source of estrogen in the body. This deleterious effect of estrogen on breast cancer is not found in women who are at least ten years beyond menopause. As a matter of fact, quite the reverse is true. In these patients, estrogens will produce a striking reduction in the size of the tumor, healing of skin ulcerations, and even disappearance of cancer in the lungs and bone.

Breast cancer discovered during pregnancy or immediately after delivery gravely alters the hope for survival. The dissemination of the disease, frequently through the bloodstream, is augmented by the "hyperhormonal," that is, increased estrogen and progesterone, state of pregnancy. Even if breast cancer has already been treated, most physicians will suggest that the patient avoid pregnancy for at least five years. Obviously, the Pill cannot be used in these patients. But if the cancer was localized at the time of surgery and if the lymph nodes in the armpits were free of tumor, many obstetricians and gynecologists would permit pregnancy after a five-year interval. One might suggest that the Pill might be utilized in such patients since the amounts of estrogen and progestin given would be minute in comparison to those occurring during pregnancy.

Although many physicians withhold the Pill from women with benign cysts of the breast (chronic cystic mastitis), I have not done so. As a matter of fact, many patients secure relief from the breast pain that occurs after ovulation by administration of one of the more androgenic oral contraceptives. Since there is no evidence that estrogen *causes* breast cancer, it is difficult to theorize that the Pill, which contains an estrogen and an anti-estrogenic progestin, might induce cancer in patients with chronic cystic mastitis.

However, if surgery is performed to remove the cysts and some tendency toward malignancy is demonstrated, I do not administer the Pill. On the basis of the diminished incidence of breast cancer in castrated women, one might theorize that this tendency toward cancer might be prevented by removing the body's estrogen or at least negating it. This is now possible because of the availability of Depo-Provera, a very potent progestin. This preparation, given once a month by injection, suppresses the ovaries to such a degree that only small amounts of estrogen are secreted. This type of management is particularly helpful to women who have large breasts with extensive cystic disease and in whom cyclic breast pain is a serious annoyance. The diminished estrogen and progesterone secretion results in reduced size of the cysts, a generalized softening of the tissues, and relief of discomfort. This treatment is usually continued for one year, and then, because of the prolonged action of the drug, ovarian estrogens are held at a low level for at least another year, sometimes longer.

CANCER OF THE ENDOMETRIUM

There have been numerous studies that suggest that a preponderance of estrogen is a factor in causing cancer of the endometrium, the third most common female cancer, ranking behind the breast and the cervix. These studies indicate that long-continued and uninterrupted estrogen may lead to a condition called *hyperplasia,* an overgrowth of the endometrium, which subsequently may become cancer *in situ* and then invasive cancer. A recent study by Dr. Saul Gusberg indicated that about 10 per cent of patients with "atypical hyperplasia" developed cancer of the endometrium if no therapy was given.[34]

Although it cannot be shown precisely that estrogen actually causes endometrial cancer, the suspicion still exists. The evidence usually cited is what I call "suggestoid" and is based on what scientists call "retrospective" data. This means that a clinical study is initiated with patients who already have cancer of the endometrium. They are then analyzed from the viewpoint of *previous* factors that *might* have predisposed these women to develop cancer. As you might expect, so many variables exist that the conclusion "cancer of the endometrium is *caused* by estrogen" is not scientifically valid. To reach this conclusion, *prospective* studies are needed. Such studies, properly randomized, are difficult, if not impossible, to program. Dr. Roy Hertz, of the National Institutes of Health, has estimated that a sample of 160,000 women of Pill-taking age, would have to be carefully evaluated for four years to detect a twofold incidence of this malignancy. Even if this were shown to be true in regard to estrogen administration, it would not necessarily follow that the same increased incidence would occur if an *estrogen plus progestin* Pill was given.

What is the evidence in favor of estrogen being the sole culprit causing this malignancy? First, we must examine two basic premises: (1) *estrogen, given in adequate doses and for a sufficiently long period of time, will produce hyperplasia;* and (2) *the presence of hyperplasia predisposes the individual to cancer.* If both are true, then we may conclude that estrogen causes cancer. There is no doubt about the validity of the first statement; the second statement is unproved. The number of patients with hyperplasia is astronomical, the number with cancer a minute fraction. Why? The hyperplasia may be temporary and the mere process of ovulation, and the effect of progesterone, reverses the process. The patient may enter menopause and her estrogen level drops precipitously. Probably the most common intervening factor is hysterectomy. Suppose 1,000 patients have endometrial hyperplasia and 900 have a hysterectomy because of the associated abnormal bleeding. Obviously, the number of women who might have developed cancer will never be known.

I attempted to find out how many women who had cancer *in situ* of the endometrium, diagnosed by curettage at the Boston Hospital for Women, subsequently developed invasive cancer. The answer—none. Of 220 patients with this diagnosis, 200 had a hysterectomy, 10 were followed for over five years and 10 were lost to follow-up.

The "suggestoid" evidence is based, in part, on the production of endometrial cancer in experimental animals who were given large doses of estrogen for prolonged periods of time. The evidence in the human is even less convincing. As far back as 1936, the late Dr. Emil Novak of Johns Hopkins Medical School in Baltimore suggested, but offered no proof, that estrogens, under certain circumstances, might cause cancer of the endometrium. Novak and several other authors noted that women having ovarian tumors that secreted large amounts of estrogen had an unusually high incidence of endometrial cancer. But other equally brilliant investigators did not find this to be so in their clinical analyses. They stated that "Neither hyperplasia nor prolonged estrogen stimulation is associated with endometrial cancer other than on a chance basis." Dr. Arthur T. Hertig, professor of pathology at Harvard Medical School, has said that "no convincing studies are available to show that estrogen stimulation alone will produce endometrial cancer, and many excellent estrogen studies fail to mention such changes as carcinoma *in situ* as occurring with regularity."[35]

Perhaps some of our own experiments in rabbits will clarify the dilemma. We were able to produce cancer in the endometrium of the rabbit, but only by using a potent cancer-producing chemical placed in direct contact with the uterine lining. If we removed the ovaries, however, the cancer did not develop. This suggests that a specific substance, such as a carcinogen, perhaps a virus, or even a predisposition of an individual, is needed to *induce* the cancer in the estrogen "primed" area. It is of interest that when we gave these rabbits a progestin such as Depo-Provera, they were protected against the development of the cancer.

What is the evidence against estrogen being the *cause* of endometrial cancer? Most women who develop this malignancy have not been taking estrogen. But this does not exclude their own ovarian estrogen as being the cause. This is true, but we have seen patients with endometrial cancer who have had their ovaries removed many years before the tumor was discovered. Furthermore, if the use of estrogenic substances *caused* this cancer, an increased incidence of this disease should now be evident, since more than thirty years have elapsed since this hormone was made available. Of course, there are more patients now with endometrial cancer, but this increase is relative to the increased population and the larger number of older women in the population. The *absolute* incidence has not changed.

Another bit of factual evidence is available in the studies of women with osteoporosis. The accepted treatment for this disease includes estrogen, calcium, and exercise. Two researchers, Drs. Wallach and Henneman, reported that only 7 patients of 242 treated with estrogen for prolonged periods developed cancer of the cervix, uterus, or ovary.[32] Not one patient in this group developed breast cancer. Six of the seven cancers in this series developed prior to 1948 when estrogen was administered continually. Only one cancer, a carcinoma *in situ* of the cervix, occurred between 1948 and 1958 when estrogen was given in cycles of twenty days each month. In another series of patients with osteoporosis treated by estrogen therapy, Gordon reported that in one thousand patient years, not one cancer of the breast, cervix, or endometrium was found. In this series, the estrogen was also given in cyclic fashion.

How does this discussion of estrogen relate to the Pill? Stated bluntly, it is impossible for the endometrium to develop hyperplasia while the Pill is being taken. The synthetic progestins in the various brands are anti-estrogenic. The endometrium eventually becomes atrophied or markedly thinned. A thin endometrium is not an ideal spawning area for cancer!

In 1959, I described the dramatic effects of various progestins on endometria showing excessive overgrowth, hyperplasia, and cancer *in situ*.[2] During progestin therapy, the endometrium is at first converted into a normal-appearing structure. But after prolonged treatment it undergoes atrophy. One of our most exciting observations occurred when we gave progestins to women with far-advanced endometrial cancer. Many of these patients were moribund from tumors in the lungs, abdomen, and pelvis. Amazing improvements followed in over one-third of these women; some are still alive years later. The progestins used in treating cancer or cancer *in situ* of the endometrium are Depo-Provera and Delalutin, two particularly potent progestins with properties very similar to natural progesterone. These compounds are now the accepted treatment for widespread endometrial cancer and are now used throughout the world. In the field of gynecological cancer it may be considered as an important breakthrough in the medical or hormonal management of malignancy.

It seems logical, at least to me, that if progestins are capable of producing a remission of endometrial cancer even when it has spread to other parts of the body, then the progestin component of the Pill might prevent or retard the development of the disease. Dr. Roy Hertz of the National Institutes of Health opposes this opinion, saying, "We must recall that practically all known carcinolytic [effective against cancer] agents, such as x-ray and certain alkylating agents, are also carcinogenic [cancer causing]." In my opinion, this may be true, but Dr. Hertz seems to be stretching a point. I know of no evidence in animals or the human female which suggests that progesterone or the synthetic progestins have *produced* endometrial cancer.

CANCER OF THE CERVIX

The second most common type of cancer peculiar to women, cancer of the cervix, differs from cancer of the endometrium and breast in that it demonstrates no response whatsoever to estrogens or progestins. Attempts to treat this disease with hormones have been uniformly unsuccessful. Although the normal cervix does respond to changes in the hormonal milieu, the malignant counterpart is totally resistant. Thus, in my opinion, cancer of the cervix is neither caused by the Pill nor is there evidence that the Pill affords direct protection against its development.

But the Pill does offer an indirect method of prophylaxis against cervical cancer. This method depends on a regular visit every six months to a physician. At this visit, examination of the breasts, cervix, uterus, ovaries, and rectum is performed. A Pap test is done at least once annually and more often if indicated.

This is a distinct advantage, for Dr. Paul A. Younge of the Boston Hospital for Women has stated that cancer of the cervix is a preventable disease if detected in its very early stages.[6] In my practice, I have diagnosed carcinoma *in situ* of the cervix in at least half-a-dozen patients who visited me for the precise purpose of obtaining the Pill. If physicians write prescriptions for only a six- or seven-months' supply of oral contraceptives, the six-month checkup will be automatic.

Dr. Gerald C. Mueller, Professor of Oncology at the University of Wisconsin and an international authority on causes of cancer, has stated, ". . . the data really argue for the fact that estrogens of their own accord are not primary carcinogens [cancer-causing]. I, personally, do not regard the threat of estrogens being carcinogenic as a very serious one."

In my opinion, the fears that the Pill might cause cancer are unjustified. Certainly the evidence available at present does not justify the repeated publicity given to this matter. There is no doubt, however, that continuing observations on the human subject are essential before final and valid conclusions may be drawn. In the meantime, the indirect advantages of the Pill in the prevention and early detection of cancer should be emphasized.

15. The Pill and Blood Clots

The LATEST medical report to spawn a series of scare stories about the Pill came from the *British Medical Journal* in its issue of April 27, 1968. It published two reports indicating a "strong relation" between oral contraceptives and death due to blood clots. These British observations were featured in newspapers and magazines and received wide radio and television coverage throughout the United States. The data was released to the news services, radio, and television at least two weeks before physicians in the United States were able to obtain the actual medical report. A typical headline appeared in *Newsweek*: PERILS OF THE PILL. The substance of this and other news reports indicated that Pill taking increased the risk of dying from blood clots in the lung or brain sevenfold.

But, with few exceptions, the news reports based on the British articles were incompletely recounted and inadequately analyzed. It seems appropriate to begin this chapter by recapitulating exactly what the English findings were.

Behind the current discussion lie two reports. One by Dr. William H. Inman, senior medical officer of the Committee on Safety of Drugs in London, and Dr. Martin P. Vessey of the Medical Research Council's statistical unit.[11] They found a "strong relation" between the use of oral contraceptives and death from pulmonary embolism (blood clots that reach the lungs) or cerebral thrombosis (blood clots in the veins of the brain) in women who did not have any condition which might have predisposed them to develop such accidents. The mortality rate per year for users of the Pill between twenty and thirty-four years of age was given as 1.5 per 100,000 and for those aged thirty-five to forty-four, 3.9 per 100,000. These figures represent approximately seven times the mortality rate from the same conditions among nonusers.

Death from coronary thrombosis (clots reaching the heart) did not appear to be linked with use of the Pill, nor did the risk of thromboembolism seem associated with any particular contraceptive.

In the second report in the same issue of the *Journal,* Dr. Vessey and Dr. Richard Doll, a co-worker in the Medical Research Council's statistical unit, investigated married women aged sixteen to forty who were discharged from nineteen large hospitals during 1964 to 1966 with a diagnosis of blood clots in the legs or lungs.[12] None of them had predisposing conditions that might have caused the clots to form. For comparison, the researchers studied married patients admitted to the same hospitals with acute surgical or medical conditions and matched them with the affected patients for age, number of children, etc. They found that of fifty-eight patients with leg or lung clots, twenty-six (45 per cent) had been using oral contraceptives during the month preceding the onset of their illness. Only 10 of the 116 "control" women (9 per cent) had been using the Pill. From these data, the researchers calculated that "The risk of hospital admission for blood clots is about nine times greater in women who use oral contraceptives" than in those who do not.

Several comments may be of interest regarding the second study. First, the total number of patients studied seems unusually small. Undoubtedly, statisticians have approved this sample as being significant, but I wonder if an incidence of 45 per cent Pill takers would have been found if one thousand or ten thousand patients were observed instead of fifty-eight. Secondly, I have been impressed by the great number of phone calls and office visits due to leg cramps, leg pain, and leg swelling by women taking the Pill. All of these women sincerely believed they had a blood clot in a vein because they had been reading about blood clots. The factor of patient awareness alone could lead to an increase in hospitalizations.

Although these new reports provide a significant statistical association between oral contraceptives and an increased incidence of thromboembolic disease, I would emphasize that the risks in the use of oral contraceptives must be weighed against the much greater risk of psychological and physical consequences of fear of pregnancy, of unwanted pregnancy, and of illegal abortion. The new evidence emphasizes the hazard of contraceptive pills for women with a history of previous blood clots or with a predisposition to blood vessel disease, as in diabetes, high blood pressure, and markedly elevated cholesterol. These women should be advised to use topical contraceptive devices.

Table III illustrates the comparative risks from oral contraceptives, pregnancy, motor accidents, and cancer in the two age groups in England, based on the *British Medical Journal* study:

TABLE III

Death Rate Per 100,000 Healthy, Married Females

	AGE	
	20–34	35–44
Pulmonary or Cerebral Emboli		
Users of Oral Contraceptives	1.5	3.9
Nonusers	0.2	0.5
Pregnancy (all risks)	22.8	57.6
Motor Accidents	4.9	3.9
Cancer	13.7	70.1
All Causes	60.1	170.5

British Medical Journal, April 27, 1968.

If full credence is given to the British findings, Pill users have a sevenfold increased risk of death due to blood clots of the lungs or brain than nonusers—and this has been emphasized in press reports. Somewhat less emphasized is the fact that these risks are extremely slight, 1.5 deaths per 100,000 in a woman twenty to thirty-four years of age, and 3.9 per 100,000 in a woman thirty-five to forty-four years of age. As shown in Table III, a British woman runs as great or greater risk when she rides in an automobile or crosses the street. Her chances of death from cancer are certainly greater. One physician expresses the degree of risk—and the degree of importance he attaches to the British findings—in this way: "For a woman under age 35, the decision to take the Pill for one year carries about the same hazard as the decision to hop into a car and drive for 12.5 miles." His comparison is based on traffic accident figures from the U. S. National Safety Council.

The comparative risk of death during pregnancy is clearly shown in Table III. The risk of death in pregnancy is seventeen times that associated with pill taking, 22.8 per 100,000 from ages 20–34 and 57.6 per 100,000 from ages 35–44. Since the Pill is the only 100 per cent effective means of contraception presently available (surgical procedures excluded), the British study clearly shows that a woman of that country has a much greater risk of death during pregnancy than by preventing it with the Pill. Furthermore her chance of dying during pregnancy from a blood clot is 1.3 per 100,000 if she is between 20 and 34 years of age—about the same as pill taking.

The British studies have been extremely valuable. They have provided a statistical basis for an impression described by numerous gynecologists and a statement made in 1962 by Dr. John Rock: "It's a lot safer to take the Pill than to be pregnant." The reports have indicated the need for further study. An editorial comment in the *British Medical Journal* reflected a typical conservative viewpoint, "While there is no cause for alarm, neither is there room for complacency." A spokesman for the British Committee on Safety of Drugs, which sponsored the research, said his group *does not* recommend withdrawal of the Pill from public use, since it has "a social and therapeutic value and is available only on prescription."

The FDA, reacting to the British study, called a meeting of major manufacturers of the Pill to discuss changes in labeling to make clear the situation as regards the Pill and embolism. The Advisory Committee on Obstetrics and Gynecology, of which Dr.

Louis M. Hellman is chairman, met with representatives of eight drug companies. The industry representatives gave the FDA their pooled data on adverse reactions to the Pill. The compilation of physician-reported adverse reactions over the past ten years showed that the incidence of death from blood clots in the lung or brain among Pill users in the United States was "well within the normal range of 0.7 to 1.6 per 100,000 per year."

The hastily summoned committee drew up a twelve-page set of guidelines for pill labeling. According to these guidelines: "Physicians should be alert to the earliest manifestations of thrombotic [blood clot] disorders. Should any of these occur or be suspected, the drug should be discontinued immediately." The difference from previous labeling reflects a *cause-and-effect* relationship between the Pill and clotting problems. Until then, the guideline used was the statement of the Advisory Committee to the FDA in 1966: "The most recent work on the response of blood coagulation factors to the oral contraceptives indicated no statistically significant effect and data derived from mortality statistics are not adequate to confirm or refute the role of oral contraceptives in thromboembolic disease."

Dr. Hellman succinctly summarized the feeling of most physicians, and my own, when he commented, "There's no sense trying to hide the risk. The problem of an adverse reaction, even in the older group, is small. *The risk of thromboembolism in pregnancy is the same as that from taking the Pill, and the overall risk of death in pregnancy is considerably higher*" (my emphasis). Dr. Hellman wondered if the British results can legitimately be transferred to the United States, since the incidence of spontaneous blood clotting disorders is geographically different. It is rare in the tropics, for example.

In this regard, data from the United States is now available. In a paper, "Oral Contraceptives and Thrombophlebitis," published in the September 30, 1968, issue of the *Journal of the American Medical Association,* Victor A. Drill, M.D., Ph.D., and David W. Calhoun, B.A., indicated that the incidence of thrombophlebitis in users of oral contraceptives was .5 per 1,000 women per year; the incidence during pregnancy was the same, .5 per 1,000 women per

9 months (projected for one year to be .7 per 1,000).[13] The incidence of thromboembolism in non-pregnant women *not* using oral contraceptives was 1.0 per 1,000 women per year based on hospital admissions. The authors also noted that women with a previous history of thrombophlebitis did not have an increased incidence of recurrence of the disease if placed on oral contraceptives. Their conclusions are as follows (italics added):

1. Studies in the United States and England have established that the incidence of thromboembolic disease in non-pregnant women of childbearing age is about 1 case per 1,000 women per year (range .71 to 1.08) based on hospital admissions for this disease, and about 2.2 cases per 1,000 women per year based on visits to the physician (range 1.2 to 3).

2. Based on 379,766 pregnancies, the antepartum incidence of thromboembolic disease is 0.5 cases per 1,000 women for 9 months; projected on a one-year basis for comparative purposes, the value is 0.7.

3. Studies on the use of oral contraceptives for 50,781 women-years give an incidence of 0.5 cases per 1,000 women per year, and one English study projects a similar incidence. *These data demonstrate a rate below the normal incidence.* A second study in England, however, calculated an incidence of 4.5, but as discussed in this review, *this rate would be subject to a large sampling error and might well be consistent with other data; this study did not find any increase in the incidence of thromboembolic phenomena from 1961 to 1966 after oral contraceptives came into use.*

4. There is *no evidence to indicate that the administration of oral contraceptives to women with a history of thrombophlebitis increases the chance of a recurrence of the disease.*

5. Evaluations made in the United States *have not demonstrated an increase in the death rate from pulmonary embolism when oral contraceptives are used and the vital statistics for England and Wales have not shown an increase in the ratio of females/males dying from thromboembolic diseases since the introduction of oral contraceptives.* A recent study in England reported no effect of oral contraceptives on the number of deaths from pulmonary embolism in women *with predisposing causes* but did conclude that there was an increased risk of thromboembolic deaths due to unknown

causes if the Pill was used. This study was *not* one of direct comparison between users and non-users, but was based on the per cent of women with blood clots in the lung who used oral contraceptives versus a "control" group without embolic disease.

Other studies are under way, notably one sponsored by the FDA at the Johns Hopkins University School of Medicine in Baltimore. Its report is due this year. Meanwhile, Dr. Howard Jones of the Johns Hopkins faculty has said, "It is my impression that the new products [oral contraceptives] with lower dosage would reduce the hazard of thromboembolic disease *if it indeed exists*" (italics added). Dr. Jones stated that he has not seen a case of thromboembolism during the last three years in patients on lower dosage regimens. Nor have I.

Several other investigators have recommended use of low-dosage pills if predisposition to embolism exists. Dr. Nichols Vorys of Ohio State University has suggested that if a patient has a marked degree of stagnation of the blood in the veins of the leg or large varicose veins or has had phlebitis (inflammation of the veins) in the past, those brands that contain the smallest amount of estrogen and progestin or ones using a progestin alone be prescribed. Dr. Vorys believes that the incidence of recurrent phlebitis in patients using the smaller-dosage compounds is minimal. Several other clinical investigations of blood-clotting factors in patients using low-dosage pills showed normal values, whereas those using the higher-dosage compounds showed a definite change in clotting capacity.

An editorial accompanying the *British Medical Journal* report notes that the oral contraceptives contain a number of very different progestins, but that only two very similar estrogens are used. This fact and other evidence that estrogens may have an effect on blood clotting, suggest that the estrogens, rather than the progestins, are responsible for the thrombosis. If this is proven to be true, there are three possible conclusions: (1) the sequential type of oral contraceptives may be more dangerous than the newer mini-dose combined pills because they contain more estrogen; (2) the continuous low-dosage progestins now under development may afford a means of avoiding thromboembolic effects since they require no estrogen; and (3) the long-term use of estrogens for any purpose—not just contraception—should be considered risky. Yet, and this is the incongruous aspect, estrogens have been used regularly for thirty years without any correlation with pulmonary or cerebral blood clots. Medical journals have published articles showing certain abnormalities in clotting mechanisms in patients taking estrogen, but no one has ever noted an increase in the thromboembolic diseases. And, since the age group receiving estrogens is usually over thirty-five, one would have expected an increase in the hormonally treated patients.

Returning to the recent British studies, information is not as yet available regarding the dose of estrogen in the Pills used. If the usual .1 mg. estrogen dose was the regimen, it is obvious that the study should be repeated using the .05 mg. estrogen pill.

The newest reports have encouraged physicians to observe caution when prescribing the Pill to patients with varicose veins, a history of phlebitis, or abnormal blood clotting. This is not to say that such patients should be denied the Pill, although previous phlebitis and pulmonary embolism are listed as contraindications. On the contrary, this may be a patient who needs protection the most. Another pregnancy carries the risk of a fatal blood clot, while the risk of the Pill is one-seventeenth that of pregnancy. In patients having a predisposition to embolism, I discuss the risks involved. A major factor to be considered is the success she and her husband have had in preventing pregnancy with condoms, diaphragms, or intrauterine devices. Tubal ligation or vaginal hysterectomy may be considered, but this necessitates surgery. Most patients are rather quick to respond that other methods of contraception have not been 100 per cent effective in their hands. Considering the much greater risks of death during pregnancy, they elect to use the Pill.

Additional fuel has recently been thrown on the blood clot fire by the report of a team of doctors at Danbury Hospital in Connecticut. They studied forty-one women on the Pill and twenty-nine women who were not, by a technique known as "lung scanning." Women in both groups had had various complaints such as coughing, leg pain, palpitation, dizziness, fever, chest pain, even coughing up blood. X-rays of the chest were not helpful in making a diagnosis. Each of these women was then given an intravenous injection of a solution containing radioactive iodine, then placed under a high-powered machine called a Magnascanner or Dynapix. The machine then measured the radioactive rays so that areas of "slowing" or "clogging" of blood in small vessels were easily detected. Twenty-two of the forty-one takers showed abnormal scans, whereas only twelve of twenty-nine nonusers exhibited the same picture. The immediate conclusion might be that the Pill causes more sludging of blood in the lungs. But Dr. Joseph L. Belsky, Assistant Clinical Professor of Medicine at Yale Medical School, commented, "The study in no way shows that the Pill is not relatively safe for the majority of women. We studied only women with symptoms, and the evidence as yet suggests that only a very small percentage of Pill users are symptomatic." Dr. Belsky suggests that any woman taking the Pill should have a scan done if she develops any of the symptoms noted above. Dr. Louis Hellman stated, "The Danbury study is interesting, but whether it has any bearing on the small amount of risk in Pill use is questionable. I'm not terribly surprised by the results. The patients' groups were unmatched, the exact denominator of the groups unknown, and the discarding of nine patients with abnormal scans in the 'control' group as compared to three in the larger Pill group seems strange." A Johns Hopkins physician, an authority on nuclear medicine, commented that the results of scanning are not always clear. "Scanning is a viable means of detecting at least the larger emboli," he noted, "but I doubt that the Danbury group can be sure of seeing the smaller emboli in smaller vessels—which they believe they are seeing."

It must be emphasized that although the British studies have established a minimal causal link between the Pill and embolism, unwarranted conclusions should not be accepted without thorough investigation. An incident that seems appropriate in this light occurred in a large planned-parenthood clinic where two women were given prescriptions for oral contraceptives. For various reasons, neither started the Pill right away, but elected to begin taking them the following month. During the month both women developed phlebitis for the first time. If these women had begun taking the pills immediately, as expected, the assumption would have been that the medication caused the phlebitis.

It is not my intention to minimize the possible dangers of the Pill's causing emboli. Extensive study is needed to determine if the low-dose pill has this effect and, if so, what ingredients in the Pill are at fault. Certainly, patients with a predisposition to clotting difficulties need to be watched very closely or another form of contraception substituted.

In the *science* of medicine certain generalizations may be made by statistical data; but in the *practice* of medicine, each patient is an individual and generalizations are not always applicable. No two patients are exactly alike and in the interest of optimum medical care, every patient must be observed as an individual and appropriate therapy prescribed.

The most perplexing problem of blood clots and the Pill will not be solved until (1) reliable rates of various blood-clotting phenomena are determined in general and specific populations; (2) laboratory tests and results are standardized; (3) common definitions of terms are agreed upon; (4) record-collection forms and data-processing techniques are developed; and (5) a large stable population is found that can be subjected to meticulous, prospective, long-range analysis.

III

THE PILL AND WOMEN'S DISORDERS

16. A Pill for Menstrual Disorders

I N ADDITION to being an effective contraceptive, the Pill has been of exceptional value in the treatment of many disorders of menstruation which have long plagued the human female. Unfortunately, this fact has been overshadowed by the furor created by the physiological, psychological, and social implications associated with use of the Pill for conception control. A few excellently documented articles have appeared describing the beneficial effects of estrogen-progestin combinations on the severity and frequency of menstrual disorders. But articles citing complications in Pill users when this medication is used for specific gynecologic problems are almost unheard of. This is incongruous, since the incidence of thrombophlebitis, eye disorders, or migraine should be just as high in this group of patients. There is another possibility. If a medication is being given for an endocrine disorder or a pelvic disease, a "normal and healthy" female is not being subjected to a medication which produces an "abnormal state." In any event, the "scare" stories and headline news rarely, if ever, report complications in these patients. But remember, the medication is exactly the same.

It is a well-worn saying that if men had babies, something would have been done to make childbirth a less painful and more enjoyable process. There is another painful and occasionally miserable process, peculiar to women, which occurs with far more monotonous regularity than childbirth, that women cannot choose to avoid, and about which men are even more ignorant and unsympathetic. I refer to the process of menstruation and its undesirable side effects that affect women prior to, during, and after this process.

Physicians have known for years that the use of estrogen alone, taken for twenty days each month to suppress ovulation, would relieve dysmenorrhea (painful menstruation) in almost 100 per cent of women. As a matter of fact, when I first began prescribing the Pill, it was not for the purpose of conception control, but for the treatment of menstrual irregularity and endometriosis. The FDA approved the Pill for these uses several years before its approval as an oral contraceptive agent.

A host of disorders revolving around ovulation and menstruation have been satisfactorily treated by the estrogen-progestin combinations. These include abnormal bleeding problems, called dysfunctional uterine bleeding, and even the total absence of menstruation, called "amenorrhea." Some women have marked irregularities in their cycles and the Pill uniformly corrects this condition, if it is due to a functional disturbance, that is, abnormal function of the ovaries. In addition, the problems of painful menstruation, painful breasts, secretion of the nipples, and the little-understood syndrome of "premenstrual tension" respond effectively to the administration of estrogen-progestin compounds.

Even such unusual disturbances as the appearance of menstrual periods and breast development in little girls from ages six to ten may be treated by the administration of progestins. The excessive bleeding that occurs in the teenage girl is due to her inability to ovulate regularly. A temporizing effect is obtained by the use of an estrogen-progestin for three to six months. After time has been gained, and anemia corrected, the process of ovulation begins, rhythm is established, and regular menses occurs. At the opposite end of the menstrual spectrum, women entering menopause experience a galaxy of symptoms due to estrogen insufficiency.

Again, the basic problem is lack of regular ovulation, and the irregular bleeding is due to an inadequate amount, or unpredictable secretion, of progesterone. Thus treatment of many women in the "premenopausal" state can be markedly improved by the Pill.

Primitive societies placed many strange taboos on women during menstruation, and it seems that we have our own taboos even in the enlightened twentieth century. Menstruation is just about the only topic now considered indelicate. Homosexuality and contraception are discussed frankly in mixed company, in the theater, and even on television. A girl can be depicted as attempting to induce an abortion, but as far as I know, discussion of menstruation, either normal or abnormal, is relegated to scientific panels or "talk shows" interviewing a physician. Menstruation has an ostrich-like effect on everyone—let's bury the subject and forget it!

Although men consider menstruation a necessary bodily function, they are delighted they don't have to bother with it. Like all bodily functions, it can be inconvenient or even a nuisance, but most women consider it a necessary, physiological phenomenon. However, a girl who has to take a day or two off from work every month because of acute abdominal pain would certainly disagree with this impression. A mother whose nerves are on edge, who drops things, forgets to order the proper groceries, who is unnecessarily cross with her children for two or three days before her period would also disagree.

Advances have been made in the field of gynecology, but none approach the magnitude of relief afforded women from menstrual difficulties by using estrogen-progestin combinations. Three major problems, properly classified as "menstrual disorders," warrant discussion. They are: (1) irregular and profuse bleeding, called "dysfunctional" bleeding, since it is due to irregular or totally absent ovulation, an abnormal *function* of the ovary; (2) painful menstruation; and (3) premenstrual tension.

IRREGULAR AND PROFUSE BLEEDING

One of the major advantages of the estrogen-progestin combinations as an oral contraceptive is the clocklike regularity of the menstrual flow. Of equal importance is the fact that the amount of menstrual bleeding is frequently less than previously experienced. One of my first papers on the Pill, presented in 1958, summarized the use of estrogen-progestin combinations in the treatment of irregular and profuse bleeding. Prior to 1955, the management of patients having dysfunctional bleeding was most unsatisfactory and required frequent curettages of the uterus and, unfortunately, many hysterectomies. Occasionally this was necessary in women in their twenties and early thirties prior to completing their childbearing potential. A tragic therapeutic measure, indeed!

In the United States and the United Kingdom, most girls begin to menstruate around the age of thirteen or fourteen. Frequently, the bleeding is irregular and profuse, particularly if a long interval occurs between periods. The basic problem is lack of ovulation and characteristically the bleeding episodes are painless. After ovulation has been established, a regular menstrual pattern develops and reproductive life is initiated. In most women the process of ovulation continues more or less regularly for about thirty years. Between ages forty-two and forty-five, the ovaries undergo an aging process, so that ovulation becomes irregular. The usual menstrual pattern at this time, the so-called premenopause, is that of skips and delays of flow. Although many women believe that any type of irregular bleeding may occur during the premenopausal period, this is not so. The misconception has been responsible for the progression of undiagnosed cancer of the cervix or the body of the uterus. After the age of fifty or fifty-two, the menstrual periods cease completely, and if menstruation does not occur for twelve consecutive months, the patient is said to be "postmenopausal."

Although most women believe that the menstrual cycle lasts precisely twenty-eight days, numerous clinical studies have indicated that women do not demonstrate such precision. Since it takes about seven days for the follicle to mature in the ovary and, following ovulation, another fourteen days (the life span of the corpus luteum if pregnancy does not occur) is needed to produce changes in the lining of the womb, the shortest ovulatory cycle is about twenty-one days. Some women have a twenty-one- or twenty-three-day cycle and for them this is perfectly normal. Others may have mild degrees of prolongation to thirty-two to thirty-five days. This is explained by the fact that in these women the follicle takes a little longer to mature. Thus, in these patients it may take twenty days for follicular maturation and their cycles would approximate thirty-four to thirty-five days. (Remember that the length of time for the follicle to develop to maturity is variable but, after ovulation, the interval to menstruation is always fourteen to sixteen days.)

Menstrual periods may be heavy or light, short or long, painful or painless, associated with extreme psychic symptoms or hardly noticed at all. I reiterate that all women experience occasional irregularities in their menstrual cycles. Dr. John Rock once said that there is nothing so regular about a woman's menstrual cycle as its irregularity. However, women who ovulate regularly have some sort of rhythm, whereas those who do not ovulate or who ovulate irregularly have no rhythm whatsoever.

As long as the menstrual flow is not excessive, scanty, painful, or associated with other disturbing symptoms, and as long as it comes in some sort of rhythmic sequence, no treatment is indicated. Skipped periods are common during adolescence and during the premenopause. Delay in establishing the menstrual cycle also occurs normally, to a certain extent, during the first three to six months following delivery of a baby. Other delays of menstruation beyond three or four consecutive months warrant investigation.

The diagnosis of dysfunctional uterine bleeding refers to any type of abnormal uterine bleeding that occurs in the absence of organic disease. Thus, the physician must exclude generalized disease states such as malnutrition, tuberculosis, excessive weight gain, excessive weight loss, and certain specific diseases of the elements of the blood. Many times it is necessary for him to perform a uterine curettage to exclude the presence of fibroid tumors or soft fleshy polyps that may grow in the interior of the womb. Occasionally, abnormal bleeding is due to other disease processes in the pelvis, such as endometriosis or pelvic infection. Having excluded these causes, the physician may then treat the abnormal bleeding. This is presently accomplished by the use of the Pill, *given in the same dosage and the same sequence as when it is used for oral contraception.* If the abnormal bleeding is not controlled by the estrogen-progestin combination, the physician should strongly suspect that a specific disease is present and that its diagnosis has been missed.

An occasional heavy period should not be of concern, but recurrent heavy bleeding at the time of the normally expected period is strongly suggestive of a fibroid growing in the womb. Intermittent bleeding throughout the cycle is always abnormal and should be investigated by curettage. However, in some patients a small amount of bleeding occurs coincident with ovulation. This is the so-called "mid-month stain" and needs no specific treatment. The patient should note that it really occurs at mid-cycle and perhaps is associated with one-sided pelvic pain, the so-called "mittelschmertz."

Staining after intercourse or douching is very suggestive of disease of the cervix. This may be simply an erosion or polyp, but it also may be due to early cancer of the cervix and should be investigated thoroughly.

Some patients will note passage of small blood clots with the menstrual period, and these are of no significance. Large clots suggest bleeding without ovulation or the presence of a fibroid. Ordinarily menstrual blood does not clot, but if it flows too freely, the factors which prevent clotting are ineffective.

To reiterate, certain types of bleeding are definitely abnormal. They should not be disregarded, and they demand that the patient see her physician so that adequate diagnosis and treatment may be initiated. These are: (1) repeatedly profuse or prolonged periods, especially if they last over seven days; (2) unexpected and irregular bleeding between periods; (3) bleeding after intercourse or douching; and (4) bleeding after menopause.

In order to make an adequate diagnosis the physician takes a complete history and performs a careful pelvic examination. In addition, he takes a Pap smear, which aids in the diagnosis of cancer of the cervix. It is important to remember, however, that cancer of the endometrium is detected by this method in only about 50 per cent of the cases. In younger individuals, the physician may elect to secure a fragment of the womb lining in the office rather than resort to curettage, which requires hospitalization and anesthesia. Subsequent treatment will depend upon the findings on pelvic examination, the Pap smear, and the endometrial tissue. Occasionally, an x-ray of the cavity of the uterus, known as a hysterogram, may be performed to note an irregularity of contour which may be produced by a polyp or a fibroid.

When the menstrual flow is excessive or prolonged, a fibroid should always be suspected. However, if a D. and C. is performed and no abnormality is discovered, the cause of the excessive bleeding is probably malfunction of the ovaries. Frequently, the curettage will produce a temporary "cure" and no further treatment is necessary. However, in many patients, abnormal bleeding will reoccur in a few months. The treatment then is quite simple. These patients are placed on an estrogen-progestin combination, daily for twenty days each month. The resulting flow is regularly spaced and normal in amount or even scanty.

If recurrent premenstrual staining is the complaint, the physician may surmise that the cause is an insufficiency of both estrogen and progesterone. Relief from this complaint is rapidly obtained by administration of an estrogen-progestin combination for seven to ten days prior to the anticipated onset of flow.

In patients who note excessive or grossly irregular bleeding, the usual cause is lack of ovulation. If the patient desires a child, the ideal treatment is induction of ovulation, usually by administration of one of the newer drugs such as Clomid or Pergonal. Subsequent to induced ovulation, normal amounts of estrogen and progesterone are secreted and the menstrual cycles become regular and normal. If, however, the patient is not married or does not wish to become pregnant, adequate treatment may be accomplished by giving estrogen-progestin combination, the Pill, in twenty-day cycles for a minimum period of six months. This results in normal episodes of bleeding, usually a scanty flow, and prevents the abnormal stimulation of the endometrium by estrogen which might cause hyperplasia. It is obvious that attempts should be made to determine why ovulation does not occur and to correct the difficulty. But regulation of menstruation and prevention of excessive bleeding may be accomplished by the Pill, even if precise factors are not immediately obvious. This is believed to be of prophylactic importance, since it has been shown that many patients who develop cancer of the endometrium have had prolonged periods of estrogen stimulation (from their nonovulating ovaries) without the protective influence of progesterone. In other words, regular ovulation and menstruation may prevent this type of cancer.

PAINFUL PERIODS

Another very definite advantage noted by women using the Pill is the disappearance of pain with the menstrual flow. This condition is known to physicians as "primary dysmenorrhea" and implies that no organic disease is present. This pain is usually crampy and located just above the pubic bone. The patient frequently complains of associated nausea, backache, legache, and generalized malaise.

The characteristic symptom, cramps, continues for twelve to fourteen hours. Patients have described their pain to me quite realistically. "It's as if," said a sixteen-year-old biology student, "the womb was doing its level best to expel the menstrual blood through a tightly closed and unwilling cervix." She said further, "As soon as the obstruction is overcome, the cramps disappear." This girl's observations are fairly close to the truth. If the cervix is widely dilated by childbirth or repeated D. and C.'s, the pain practically disappears—at least for a time. Moreover, if ovulation does not occur, painful periods are absent. Why? If only estrogen stimulates the cervix, it becomes soft and the opening dilates slightly, just as it does prior to ovulation to let the sperm through. But after ovulation, presumably due to the effect of progesterone, the cervix closes and becomes quite spastic.

Primary dysmenorrhea is a disturbance of *function* and is not a pathological condition. It is influenced by a variety of physiological and psychological events. It is more common and more severe in high-strung, nervous girls and women, especially those of excess sensitivity who tend to overreact and to whom, as a consequence of early training, the psychological import of menstruation is that of being "sick" or "unwell." The process is common in young girls whose mothers have had the same monthly disability. I have noted it to occur frequently in girls of Italian or Spanish descent; it is rare in those of Nordic extraction. In clinics frequented by Negroes, it is hardly ever seen, and during a recent visit to South Africa, I was amazed by its rarity among the Bantu.

Painful periods account for a great deal of "time off" among workers in industry and offices in the United States. Nurses at large plants are besieged by women seeking temporary relief, and personnel directors shy away from hiring potential employees who give a history of incapacitating menstrual periods. The number of hours lost from work due to this disorder must be astronomical.

The cause of painful periods is unknown, but it is assumed to be due to degeneration of the endometrium after ovulation, with subsequent sloughing of this tissue. A tightly closed cervix may aggravate the process. Subsequently, the muscle of the uterus undergoes excessive activity and a true muscle cramp, similar to that which grips the calf of the leg, may occur.

The most effective "treatment" for primary dysmenorrhea is a sympathetic, factual explanation of the menstrual process, the undoing of superstitions or resentful attitudes, such as the feeling that menstruation is a "curse" or "sickness," rather than an index of normal womanhood. Patients are encouraged to be active, to participate in sports, to carry on in a normal fashion, rather than taking to their beds for a day or two each month. But there is no single treatment for all patients. Some are relieved by mild preparations such as aspirin or Edrisal. Hot tub baths, long held to be dangerous at this time, may be comforting.

Since dysmenorrhea occurs only in ovulatory cycles, hormones have been used to suppress ovulation. I have been using estrogen for twenty-five years to do just this, suppressing ovulation for nine or ten months of each year. But the Pill accomplishes the same effect.

Numerous patients using the estrogen-progestin combinations as an oral contraceptive have noted marked improvement in the severity of uterine cramps accompanying their periods. It is believed that the newer compounds affect the process of sloughing of the endometrium and diminish the degree of contraction of the uterine muscle. If the pain associated with the menses is aggravated by the estrogen-progestin compounds, the possibility of the disease endometriosis is strongly suggested.

PREMENSTRUAL TENSION

The premenstrual syndrome, depending as it does on the process of ovulation and subsequent bleeding, is undoubtedly one of the enigmas of gynecology. Many women of childbearing age suffer from the insidious symptoms, but the exact incidence is unknown. The symptoms range from an indefinable depression and fatigue to severe migraine headaches. It is nearly always accompanied by irritability, moodiness, and bad temper.

It has been estimated that about 120 million working days a year are lost because of this disorder, and accidents in the home and on the highways are thought to increase during the premenstrual days. In one British prison, one-half of 156 newly convicted women had committed their crimes just before or during menstruation.

In a recent study, the scientific director of the medical commission on accident prevention in Great Britain stated that a survey of ten thousand working women indicated that they were accident prone a few days before and during menstruation. He cited further evidence to suggest that women *taking the contraceptive pill were not accident prone at this time.* It might seem that "taking the Pill" is a drastic solution to this problem, although many women are using estrogen-progestin combinations for less-documented disturbances such as the improvement of the skin and hair. Why, then, should it not be taken for discomfort and unhappiness?

In modern society menstruation is regarded by most women as a necessary nuisance. The variety of names for this process used by the teenagers of America indicates the distaste that most of them exhibit. If the menstrual flow is associated with pain, it is usually called "the curse," a term very similar to the primitive "possessed by demons." Another phrase is "being unwell" or "having my sick period" or even the most unusual terminology, "fallen off the roof." What these descriptions really imply is that for a few days prior to each menstrual period, a miserable set of symptoms occurs that have been grouped together in a most inadequate medical term, "premenstrual tension."

Premenstrual tension is a common process and, at one time or another, almost 70 per cent of women experience it. Yet many do not recognize the association and do not seek medical assistance. This disorder has no respect for age, although it is more common in women during their late thirties and early forties. It does not cease until a woman stops ovulating and menstruating. If there are any real blessings due to the menopause, the relief of the monthly emotional changes that plague so many women for two days to two weeks before each period must be classified as one of these.

Certain European countries regard the premenstrual tension syndrome as "temporary insanity." Women are considered less responsible for bizarre actions during this time of the month. One shoplifter exhibited her unusual tendencies only during the immediate premenstrual phase and was promptly acquitted when the judge was informed of the fact that the patient was "temporarily insane" during this time. It is interesting to note, however, that in California a woman arrested for shoplifting stated that these tendencies exhibited themselves only after she started to take the Pill. She was not acquitted.

The symptoms of premenstrual tension are varied and one or more may be present at the same time or at different intervals before and during menstruation. These include bloating, headache, fullness of the breasts, tenderness of the breasts and nipples, swelling of the ankles and feet, weight gain, abdominal discomfort or distress, backache, migraine, aggravation of acne, nervousness, insomnia, irritability, change in libido, poor concentration and, a term employed most by husbands, "bitchiness." Husbands frequently complain to gynecologists, "Doctor, please do something with my wife, she's not fit to live with at certain times of the month."

Women athletes frequently will not participate in the competitive events during the premenstrual phase, and many dancers and actresses find their performances vary from mediocre to "lousy" at this time. Singers even avoid appearances during the premenstrual phase because of voice impairments due to congestion of the vocal cords.

There are numerous theories as to the cause of premenstrual tension, but none is established in the minds of most physicians except for the swelling due to salt and water retention.

Since there is rather generalized swelling throughout the body, similar localized areas may occur in the brain. This is probably the cause of the emotional symptoms and possibly of the migraine-type headaches. Some women seem to be particularly susceptible to salt and water retention and, as mentioned previously, this is primarily an effect of estrogen. I have seen patients who tell me they gained six or seven pounds within twenty-four hours of a cocktail party where salty canapes or salted nuts were served.

The various theories advanced for the excessive edema have included: (1) an excessive amount of estrogen; (2) an abnormal relationship between estrogen and progesterone; (3) an excess of progesterone; (4) a deficiency of progesterone; (5) an excess of the pituitary hormone that prevents excretion of salt and water through the kidney; and (6) a specific allergy to either estrogen or progesterone. Although some physicians feel that psychological factors predominate in causing the marked swelling, the evidence at present suggests that the entire disorder is due to a combination of hormonal and psychic factors.

It is evident that premenstrual tension occurs only in women who ovulate, therefore, any method of ovulation suppression will prevent the symptoms. This involves the administration of agents such as the estrogen-progestin combinations for twenty days of each month. If there are other reasons for taking such a preparation, such as contraception and/or dysmenorrhea, this method of therapy is quite desirable. In addition, the swelling is reduced by administration of a diuretic taken with breakfast, usually in a regimen of three days on and three days off. This may be initiated just following ovulation or roughly about ten days prior to the expected menstrual flow. As mentioned previously, prolonged administration of a diuretic diminishes its effectiveness and may lead to excessive loss of salt and potassium, causing leg cramps and weakness. In certain patients the use of progesterone or a synthetic progestin during the last seven to ten days of the cycle may bring about marked improvement. Certain proprietary medications include a diuretic, a synthetic progestin, and a tranquilizer. I also impress upon my patients the importance of salt restriction during the premenstrual period.

A few patients, particularly those who have severe swelling of the breasts with associated pain, experience marked relief from a male hormone in small doses when given for one week after ovulation. Other investigators have found that the male hormone, given prior to ovulation, may have a salutary effect, although the amount given is inadequate to prevent ovulation.

Some of the newer oral contraceptives contain only .05 mg. of estrogen and a progestin with slight male-hormone tendencies. Such agents are quite effective in the management of breast engorgement and tenderness that accompany premenstrual tension.

17. A Pill for Women's Diseases

In THIS CHAPTER, a group of diseases will be discussed that have been shown to respond to the administration of the sex hormones, estrogen and progesterone. Research concerning these diseases gained momentum during the last decade, shortly after the newer and more potent agents became available. Outstanding advances have been made, particularly in treating endometriosis, some forms of infertility, repeated miscarriage, and premature menstruation in young girls.

ENDOMETRIOSIS

The disease known as endometriosis and its role in the history of the development of the Pill has already been discussed in Chapter 3. Briefly stated, portions of the endometrium migrate through the Fallopian tubes into the abdominal cavity where they implant on the ovaries, bladder, colon, and other ligaments that support the uterus. The errant endometrial cells continue to grow and bleed, causing painful periods, irregular bleeding, and, eventually, infertility.

Until 1955, unless the woman became pregnant, about the only effective treatment was a hysterectomy, a tragedy for the young, unmarried woman. Estrogens and male hormones had been used prior to this time and, while successful, the side effects of prolonged treatment were disturbing to many patients. Furthermore, these hormonal agents did not produce changes in areas of endometriosis that occurred during pregnancy, which was still the best treatment for the disease. My own search for an improved therapy was the spur that led to my first use of the medication that became the Pill.

Today thousands of women with endometriosis are treated by a pseudopregnancy. In this therapeutic approach, an estrogen and progestin combination is administered continually (noncyclically) for periods of six months or longer. Any contraceptive pill may be used. Over 80 per cent of the patients note improvement. The misplaced endometrial cells degenerate in the same manner that occurs during normal pregnancy. A disease which was once a tragedy and a major cause of hysterectomies in young females may now be effectively controlled by estrogen-progestin combinations.

INFERTILITY

Some years ago, Dr. John Rock suggested that the estrogen-progestin combinations might be useful in treating patients with "idiopathic infertility," that is, patients in whom no cause for their infertility could be found. Dr. Rock's experiments with such infertile women were described in Chapter 4. By creating a pseudopregnancy for several months, Dr. Rock observed that about 10 per cent of his patients subsequently became pregnant. He suggested that a "pituitary rebound" had occurred after temporary suppression of that gland. Studies by other investigators have not substantiated Dr. Rock's original observations, except in those patients having an insufficiency of the endometrium or inadequate development of the uterus. In such patients, the estrogen-progestin does seem to produce a more normal development of these reproductive organs.

It is true that most women who have previously had babies become pregnant rather quickly after the Pill is discontinued. Unfortunately, this is not so for women with prolonged infertility. If, however, the infertility is hormone-caused, estrogen-progestin combinations may be therapeutic. Physicians speak of "inadequate luteal phase," meaning that the corpus luteum either produces an insufficient amount of progesterone to prepare the endometrium for implantation of a fertilized egg or that the endometrium is particularly resistant to that hormone. The preferred treatment in such cases is to inject a pituitary-like hormone called Human Chorionic Gonadotrophin—HCG (obtained from the placenta of the human female)—soon after ovulation. The hormone stimulates the corpus luteum to secrete more estrogen and progesterone so that the lining of the womb will be better prepared to accept the fertilized egg. In some women, however, the corpus luteum apparently is inadequately developed and even stimulation by HCG is not effective. In these individuals, I have used an estrogen-progestin compound to substitute for the hormone deficiency. This is accomplished by giving the Pill for about a week, beginning three or four days after ovulation. I usually repeat this scheme for several months to "prime" the endometrium before suggesting that pregnancy be permitted.

MISCARRIAGES

The treatment with estrogen-progestin or HCG is particularly effective in women classified as "habitual aborters." This term implies that at least three consecutive spontaneous miscarriages, usually during the first twelve weeks of pregnancy, have previously occurred. My method of treating these patients is to prevent pregnancy and simultaneously "prime" the endometrium for three or four months by giving one of the sequential oral contraceptives. At the conclusion of the artificial cycles, the patient begins to chart her basal body temperature. She may then be able to detect the time of ovulation, and intercourse is planned accordingly. The basal body temperature drops within fourteen to sixteen days after ovulation, just prior to menstruation. If the temperature remains elevated for eighteen consecutive days, pregnancy may be assumed and a potent progestin-estrogen combination, such as Deluteval, is administered to correct any hormonal insufficiency that may exist.

Many early miscarriages occur at a very critical point soon after the egg is implanted. In such cases, the women never know of their conception. They usually have what appears to them to be a delayed and heavy menstrual flow. But the conceptus is actually discarded at this time. The newer tests for pregnancy become positive about the twenty-first day after fertilization. If the test is positive, an estrogen-progestin is injected weekly until the sixteenth week of pregnancy. In many of my patients with habitual miscarriages (some with eight consecutive losses), I have found this method, together with the administration of HCG during the luteal phase, to be quite effective. Unfortunately, HCG cannot be continued for more than two or three injections, since it alone will cause the body temperature to remain falsely elevated. This is due to its effect on the corpus luteum and the continued secretion of progesterone. Remember, it is progesterone that causes the temperature rise. Moreover, since the tests for pregnancy are based on the presence of the patient's own HCG derived from the primitive cells that eventually will make up the placenta, continued injections of HCG will give a falsely positive pregnancy test.

Although the treatments just described are most useful in aiding implantation, there is no evidence these compounds will correct the abnormalities associated with a threatened miscarriage. If a patient has uterine cramps and bleeding, most gynecologists believe that progesterone or estrogens are of no value in saving the pregnancy. Actually, the hormones stop the bleeding and cramps, but the fertilized egg and its surrounding tissue degenerate. The patient is lulled into a false sense of pregnancy, whereas she is actually in a state of pseudopregnancy resulting from the estrogen-progestin she is receiving.

It is imperative, therefore, when a physician administers hormones prior to cramps and bleeding, particularly in a patient who is a habitual aborter, that he perform a pelvic examination every two or three weeks and follow the progress of the pregnancy by sequential pregnancy testing. There is no evidence to suggest that an abnormal pregnancy can be continued by use of these agents, resulting in the birth of an abnormal baby.

PREMATURE MENSTRUATION

One of the more unusual, but nonetheless striking uses of the newer progestational agents is in the treatment of precocious puberty. For unknown reasons, the pituitary begins to secrete the necessary hormones (FSH) to mature the follicle in the ovary and even to produce ovulation (with LH) in girls under the age of ten. As a result of the estrogen secreted by the growing follicle, breast development occurs, together with the appearance of pubic and axillary hair and even menstruation.

Although certain tumors of the brain and even an infection such as meningitis may cause premature menstruation, most of those so afflicted have no specific cause. Not only are the symptoms embarrassing to the child and her parents, but the estrogen secreted may affect the growth of long bones, resulting in diminished height.

One of the newer synthetic progestins, Depo-Provera, is so potent that it will suppress the hormones of the pituitary, diminish the growth of the follicle in the ovary, reduce the amount of estrogen being secreted, and prevent further bleeding and breast development. The child grows in a normal fashion. The treatment with Depo-Provera is usually continued until the time of normal adolescence.

18. Feminine Forever?
The Pill and Menopause

A N INCH-HIGH headline in *Vogue* magazine encouraged its readers to LIVE YOUNG AT ANY AGE. *McCall's* breathlessly described PILLS TO KEEP WOMEN YOUNG. In Canada, *MacLean's* wrote thousands of words about "Medicine's New Boon to Women: A PILL THAT PROLONGS THE PRIME OF LIFE." *Women's Day* in Sydney Australia, carried this report from "our New York Office"—NOW . . . BEAUTY BONUS FROM THE PILL. *Cosmopolitan* editors ecstatically penned this headline: OH WHAT A LOVELY PILL!

These are but a few of the scores of newspaper and magazine stories printed around the world to report that the Pill and ERT— Estrogen Replacement Therapy—can keep a woman "feminine forever." By ingesting hormones, particularly estrogen, a woman can stop the clock and even reverse the passage of time, foiling Nature by remaining young and beautiful and vibrant while she is practically on her way to the grave. Clearly, if I read such stories correctly, Ponce de Leon looked in the wrong time and place for the fountain of youth. He should have sent Mrs. de Leon to a modern gynecologist.

Such claims for the anti-aging effects of hormones find a ready audience, for in our present American culture youth is the keynote. The baby boom of the 1940's and 1950's has become the youth boom of the 1960's. The majority of our population is under thirty and a dominant theme of advertising is the appeal to youth. Significant numbers of women in their forties and fifties see the world passing them by and beseech their mirrors for a more positive answer to the old fairy tale question, "Who is the fairest in the land?"

Until recently, the older woman sought to restrain the march of time with longer visits to the beauty parlor, larger expenditures for cosmetics, padded bras, uncomfortable girdles, contact lenses, caps for the teeth, stringent diets, exercise machines, "nose jobs," and "face lifts." Now, the shield against time is supposed to be estrogen.

I am not unsympathetic to the plight of the older woman. There is something basically unfair in the way the two sexes age. A man ages gracefully without any major hormonal shifts, but a woman undergoes a major physiological change between the ages of forty and fifty-five years that coincide with the period of peak productiveness in most men.

Men seem to age gradually or not at all—at least until well into the sixties.[36] W. Somerset Maugham stated at his eightieth birthday party that "There are many virtues in growing old." Then, following an embarrassing pause in which the audience started to become uneasy, he added, "I'm just trying to think what they are." Maugham remained vital and productive well into old age, and so have many others, Churchill, Toscanini, Chagall, Casals, Chaplin, Casey Stengel, to name a few in a variety of professions. An equally long list of famous older women might be cited: Eleanor Roosevelt, Helen Keller, Faith Baldwin, Helen Hayes, Marianne Moore. But these women achieved beauty of soul rather than a reflection in a mirror. Perhaps the best barometer of the male advantage in aging comes from Hollywood. Veteran actors such as Cary Grant, John Wayne, James Stewart, Glenn Ford, and Henry Fonda are still playing leading men, while their female contemporaries are either retired or relegated to character parts.

It is of small comfort to a woman, but a fact nonetheless, that the human female is the only mammal whose life span exceeds the reproductive period. In every other species, the female dies when she can no longer conceive. Until a few decades ago, this was true of most women. In 1900 the average life span of a woman was forty-five years, roughly coincidental with menopause. It is also true that man continues to produce hormones, and often sperm, into extremely advanced old age, while a woman's natural production of estrogen is sharply curtailed along with her ovarian function during menopause. A better ovarian design would have separated ova from estrogen synthesis, permitting continuation of sex hormone production in the absence of developing eggs. If the only difference between male and female is the absence of sex hormone, is it logical to assume that giving estrogen to a postmenopausal woman would permit her to age just as gracefully as natural male hormones assist men?

This assumption is correct—in the main. Gynecologists have been using estrogens for thirty years or more, and there is no doubt about the subjective and objective improvement in premenopausal, menopausal, and postmenopausal patients. Whether these improvements retard the aging process is a question of semantics. At the same time, many of us are suspicious (to put it mildly) about the fantastic claims of the protagonists of the "feminine forever" school. In this chapter I will present a realistic appraisal of what I believe estrogen therapy will and will not do.

THE AGE OF MENOPAUSE

Increase in life expectancy has destined the average woman to live about twenty-five years of her life with the symptom-complex resulting from ovarian deficiency. The age at which menopause occurs does not appear to be related to the age of onset of the menses or childbearing, but it is influenced by physical, emotional, constitutional, social, and racial factors. Daughters tend to follow their mother's menstrual pattern, suggesting that menopausal age is probably determined genetically. There is a popular saying that if you want to live long, pick your ancestors wisely.

Although premature menopause may occur spontaneously any time between the ages of sixteen and thirty-five years, menstruation ceases between the ages of thirty-five and fifty in about 50 per cent of women. In American women, the average age of menopause is forty-eight years. But there has been a noticeable increase in the number of women who continue to menstruate normally through the age of fifty and over. A word of warning, however. Bleeding beyond age fifty may be interpreted by a woman as "menstruation" when it may be due to cancer of the uterus or an ovarian tumor secreting estrogen. I exhort women over the age of fifty who continue to bleed, even in regular cycles, to visit their physician so that Pap smears and biopsies may be performed.

A four-year delay, to an average age of fifty years at menopause, has occurred in British women during the past century. The increased menstrual life may be attributed to better standards of living associated with a general improvement in health and nutrition. However, it has been suggested that the delayed menopausal age may be predetermined by an increase in the number of eggs in the ovary at birth or may be due to a reduction in the rate of follicle and egg decay. As I have mentioned previously, there is no evidence that the Pill, by preventing ovulation, will store the eggs for later use. During Pill use, the eggs undergo degeneration in the same way that occurs during pregnancy.

Our population in the United States has changed considerably in the last half decade. There is no doubt that our American culture emphasizes youth, but an increasing emphasis is now being directed to the geriatric group. In the 1960 census, there were over 10,000 Americans 100 years of age or older, that is, 1 in every 17,000 persons. Biologically, the maximum span of life for humans is about 115 years, and perhaps by the year 2000 this will be our time on earth. Scientific advances have upset Nature's timetable for the female. In 1900 the life expectancy for females was 49.2 years; in 1960 it was 75.1 years. One might speculate that, as longevity increases, the span of possible fecundity might also increase. If this is so, the control of ovulation for conception control might be extended to grandmothers and even great-grandmothers.

THE PHYSIOLOGY OF MENOPAUSE

The word menopause comes from the Greek words for "month" and "cessation." The ovary ceases to secrete estrogen and the lining of the womb is no longer stimulated to grow. If a woman between the ages of forty-five and fifty-two does not menstruate for twelve consecutive months, she is said to have entered the menopause.[37]

A more comprehensive term is "climacteric," which also comes from two Greek words, one meaning "rung of a ladder" and the other "a critical time." The climacteric refers to the years during which menopause occurs, roughly ages forty to sixty. I have used the term "perimenopausal" to refer to the years just before and after menopause. By whatever terminology, it is important to remember that cessation of the menses is only one aspect in a series of physiological changes.

The hormonal structure of reproduction was reported in Chapter 3. Briefly reviewed, the ovary releases a small amount of estrogen that first stimulates the hypothalamus, and then the pituitary, to release a hormone, FSH. This hormone stimulates the follicle containing the egg to grow and mature. Another hormonal "signal" from the ovary permits the release of a second hormone from the pituitary, LH. This hormone bursts the ripened follicle, releasing the egg. Within twenty-four hours, the corpus luteum or "yellow body" develops from the ruptured follicle. The corpus luteum secretes large amounts of estrogen and progesterone, and these hormones shut off the release of FSH and LH so that further ovulation is prevented during the cycle. In addition, estrogen and progesterone prepare the endometrium for implantation of the fertilized egg.

As a woman reaches her mid-forties, aging of the ovary begins. Maturation of the follicle takes longer. Instead of the usual fourteen days needed for maturation, the follicle may require thirty or more days for this process to occur. Since menstruation occurs fourteen days after ovulation, a menstrual cycle of forty-four days results. As the aging process progresses, the cycle may extend to ninety or more days. The premenopausal woman frequently experiences highly irregular menstruation, although pregnancy may still occur. The characteristic pattern is that of skips and delays of periods—not intermenstrual bleeding.

Finally, the day comes when the follicles do not mature. They develop to a certain state then degenerate, a process known as atresia. As the ovary ages, its blood supply becomes deficient; it shrivels and shrinks, and its functioning elements are replaced by scar tissue. For all intents and purposes, the ovary is dead. The eggs are gone and the amount of estrogen secreted is minimal. But the pituitary does its level best to stimulate the aged ovary by increasing its output of FSH and LH. Measurements have shown increases to almost twenty times the normal amount. Although both FSH and LH are secreted in increased amounts, the usual burst of LH, so characteristic of ovulation, does not occur. The hormonal situation in the menopausal woman may be summarized as one of increased FSH and LH, low estrogen, and no eggs. This condition may persist for eight or ten years. The excess pituitary secretion eventually returns to normal then diminishes. Thus for the remainder of her life the human female must live in a state of estrogen insufficiency.

There are other changes of equal importance. Secretion of pituitary hormones regulating adrenal and thyroid function and even that of growth hormone are affected. The decreased estrogen is associated with a decrease in general anabolism (protein building) and this is aggravated by the continued secretion of adrenal hormones which are catabolic (protein destroying). This predominance of tissue destruction over a period of time is believed to result in some of the metabolic changes occurring in postmenopausal women. These include: protein depletion and muscle wasting, obesity, hypertension, joint pains, osteoporosis (bone degeneration), diabetes, and arteriosclerosis (hardening of the arteries). Although these disorders develop gradually, they are similar to those observed after removal of the ovaries by surgery or ovarian destruction by x-ray. The menopausal woman may be considered to be a "physiological castrate."

Before the supply of eggs has been exhausted, the process of ovulation sputters then comes to an abrupt halt. Estrogen continues to be secreted for several years, but progesterone is absent since ovulation does not occur. In my estimation, this progesterone insufficiency is of no importance. Progesterone is necessary for the establishment and maintenance of pregnancy, nothing more. Therefore, I am not in favor of its use in the postmenopausal female. The insufficiency is that of estrogen, not progesterone.

Before explaining the importance of estrogen, this point should be made: The Pill offers four distinct advantages to the premenopausal woman: (1) the estrogen and progestin suppress FSH and LH, preventing ovulation and pregnancy; (2) the menstrual cycles occur with clocklike regularity; (3) if an estrogen insufficiency exists, this may be corrected by the administration of a Pill selected specifically for its estrogen content; (4) the process of overgrowth of the endometrium (hyperplasia) and its associated profuse flowing is prevented.

But even if the premenopausal woman is taking the Pill, the process of ovarian aging continues. When she reaches age fifty or fifty-two, the ovaries have only minimal function. Ovulation becomes impossible, although in some women, not all, moderate amounts of estrogen are still secreted. When the estrogen production reaches a critically low level, symptoms and signs of hormonal insufficiency occur. It is at this point that estrogen replacement therapy is deemed advisable.

WHAT HAPPENS IN MENOPAUSE?

What are the symptoms of menopause besides the irregularities or absence of the monthly cycle? Many women begin to feel irritable and nervous. They have "hot flashes." They become emotionally unstable, weep easily, and feel insecure and inadequate to meet the demands that life makes of them. They feel depressed. They begin to lose interest in an active sex life with their husbands.

There are other serious changes. Their bodies begin to lose the firmness of skin and muscle tone of which they were so proud. Their breasts begin to shrink and become flabby; they put on weight around the waist and hips, develop jowls, and wrinkles appear on their necks and faces. Insidiously, their bones begin to become thin and brittle. They may develop high blood pressure, and their blood cholesterol may rise.

With the passage of time and the use of tranquilizing drugs, the postmenopausal female may regain her emotional balance without too much difficulty. But the aging of her body continues, now quite rapidly if her production of estrogen has ceased completely. Some women, however, continue to produce estrogen in limited amounts for ten or fifteen years after menopause, and the changes in these women are gradual.

The postmenopausal woman, according to statistics, is just as vulnerable to cardiovascular disorders as a man her own age. She may now develop high blood pressure, hardening of the arteries, and other metabolic diseases. Before menopause, women are rarely subject to these disorders. There is suggestive evidence that her continuing production of estrogen is a protection against them.

Because the lack of estrogen causes a negative protein balance in her system, protein is withdrawn from the bones and she is no longer capable of storing calcium at a proper level. Her bones gradually become even thinner and more brittle. She loses height, develops a "dowager's hump" between her shoulder blades, has back and joint pains and may develop arthritis. In addition, teeth and gum trouble may occur.

As a result of these various aches and pains, she becomes less and less active and the degenerating muscle tone deteriorates further. She has even less interest in sharing an active sex life, partly because her genital organs are shrinking and becoming dry, irritable, and even painful. She becomes more subject to vaginal infections, as well, because of these changes. Her lack of interest in physical companionship with her husband may also lead to serious family problems which further complicate her physical ailments.

Eventually, as menopause is well established, her skin becomes tougher and deeply lined. Her breasts wither. Her hair becomes coarser, but pubic and axillary hair almost disappear. The labial structures lose their supporting structure and normal lubrication. She can't seem to control the spare tire around her waist, she loses interest in her appearance and may become careless about it.

Occasionally, in a woman whose estrogen production has ceased completely, the adrenal glands increase their production of male hormone, and the woman becomes progressively masculinized. She begins to grow coarse hair on the face, arms, and legs. Her voice deepens and other changes take place that are most disturbing to a woman. She may even get bald.

EFFECTS OF ESTROGEN

The effects of estrogen are widespread throughout the body. The major ones are:

1. On hot flashes—Although the precise mechanism is unknown, estrogen sensitizes the balance between an area of the brain known as the diencephalon and the autonomic (involuntary) nervous system which regulate important body functions such as heart rate, breathing, and the motility of the stomach and intestines. Lowering of the estrogen level produces increased irritability of small blood vessels in the skin, particularly in the blush areas. When these vessels dilate, an increased blood flow occurs, resulting in a sensation of warmth. This is the so-called "hot flash." The autonomic nerves then try to regulate body temperature by release of water through the skin. Evaporation of the perspiration is a cooling process, and it is accompanied by constriction of the tiny blood vessels and lessened blood flow. This is the so-called "cold flash" of menopause.

2. On breasts—A deficiency of estrogen also produces changes in the breasts. Engorgement of breast tissue is due to salt and water retention and stimulation of mammary glands and ducts. Estrogen is responsible for both effects. When this hormonal stimulation is deficient, the breasts become soft, the supporting tissue stretches and the patient complains of sagging breasts.

3. On the genital organs—Although estrogen stimulates the growth of the uterus and development of the Fallopian tubes, its major importance in the perimenopausal female is on the lining of the vagina. The growth of the cells that permit the vagina to have a certain amount of elasticity and secretion are stimulated by estrogen. In its absence the vagina becomes a rigid, thin tube that

is totally unprepared for the act of intercourse. Furthermore, the vagina then becomes prone to infection by *Trichomonas vaginalis* (TV in the lingo of doctors) and multiple other bacteria.

The tissue that lines the vagina also extends into the urethra for a short distance. In the absence of estrogen, this lining becomes thin and easily infected by bacteria in the vagina. The result is that of burning and frequency of urination. Women may frequently lose urine in their haste to find a bathroom, a process known as "urge incontinence."

4. On hair growth—Estrogens work in synergism with male hormones (from the adrenal) in the development of axillary and pubic hair. This is illustrated in a disease state where women are born with testes instead of ovaries. The testes make both estrogens and male hormone, but the tissues of the body are peculiarly resistant to the male hormone. The resulting body type is outstandingly female with round hips and normal breast development—but *pubic and axillary hair are absent.* The hair on the scalp, however, is normal and is, therefore, not dependent on the admixture of male hormone. The beautiful, thin hair of the female is undoubtedly estrogen-related, since in tumors of the adrenal or ovary which secrete large amounts of male hormone, the thin hair becomes coarse and subsequently facial hair may become a beard.

5. On body metabolism—Primarily estrogens increase protein synthesis and aid in the deposition of a carbohydrate, glycogen, in the liver. Specific enzymes needed for the manufacture of all important cell proteins, DNA and RNA,* are dependent upon estrogen. In addition, estrogens reduce cholesterol in the blood and increase specific fatty substances known as phospholipids and lipoproteins, thus affording a protective mechanism against diseases of the arteries and coronary attacks. (In the male, androgens, male hormones, do just the opposite.) Estrogens increase water retention in tissues of the body and there is a tendency to prevent loss of calcium, although definite proof of this is lacking. At puberty, estrogens cause closure of the epiphyses, growing ends of the long bones, thus affecting the height of the female child.

---

* Desoxyribonucleic and Ribonucleic acids.

Bone density is maintained by estrogens, a most important factor in the prevention of osteoporosis.

Concluding that the way to prevent all of these undesirable effects of estrogen insufficiency is to administer estrogen either orally or by injection is like adding 2 and 2 and getting 22. Estrogen therapy, while of value to many patients, is really not that simple.

THE CLAIMS OF THE FEMININE "FOREVERISTS"

All women want to be young. All women want to be feminine. Theoretically, and according to some authorities, simply by taking the Pill women can stay forever young, forever feminine.

No pill can make a premenopausal woman youthful. Nor can estrogen make her feminine, if she is not. Estrogen will not make her gentle and charming in the womanly, wifely, motherly sense, or "girlish" in the sex-appealing, eye-appealing sense. The Pill is not related to sexual activity, nor is it a cure-all for the strains and stresses of a woman's life.

Grace Naismith, writing in the *Reader's Digest,* observed that "Thousands of women, mostly in middle age, have been caught up by the claims made for the estrogen pill. Wooed by enthusiastic articles and sensational advertisements, they have overwhelmed doctors with pleas to 'make me young again.' "[36]

The trend is becoming a matter of concern to many reputable physicians. Many women in the premenopausal period of life come to my office stating, "I am so depressed and I am getting to look so old." Most of these women are ovulating and menstruating normally and have no insufficiency of estrogen or progesterone.

The conclusions derived from the avalanche of literature on the use of estrogens in both the medical and lay press vary widely, depending upon the age, sex, and medical background of the reader. The postmenopausal woman envisions the return of youth, beauty, vigor, and sexual interest subsequent to the administration of estrogen and progestins. The premenopausal woman is ecstatic at the thought of preventing the dreaded symptoms of the menopause and the associated facial wrinkles, drooping breasts, muscular weakness, and diminished libido. The internist sees the possibility of preventing disease, particularly arteriosclerosis and osteoporosis (bone degeneration); and the psychiatrist hopes for an improved adjustment to an abrupt and dramatic change in self-concept.

The gynecologist, however, casts a suspicious glance at these fantastic claims, and rightfully so, since those of us who have been using estrogenic substances for over thirty years have not seen the extravagant improvements and prophylaxis cited by protagonists of the "Feminine Forever" school.

Rather, gynecologists are worried about breast tenderness and masses, the reappearance of fibroids of the uterus, and irregular bleeding. Some physicians, without adequate scientific proof, have associated the administration of estrogens with cancer of the breast and uterus.

Estrogens have been administered to postmenopausal, surgically castrated, prematurely menopausal, or congenitally deficient females (women born without ovaries) by most gynecologists since potent compounds became available in the 1930's. So there is really nothing new or earthshaking in the feminine-forever concept. What is all the excitement about? What is being ballyhooed is really a minor variation on an old estrogen theme. What has been done is that a few physicians have concocted a rather elaborate therapeutic scheme on the conclusions that: (1) *all* estrogen-deficient women should receive hormonal replacement unless contraindications exist; (2) medication should be continued forever; (3) estrogens should be given for a prolonged period of time (60, 90, 120 days) and interrupted occasionally with a progestin (to prevent the development of hyperplasia of the endometrium during the prolonged administration); (4) dosage should be increased or decreased as indicated by vaginal smears; (5) the intermittent use of progestin will diminish the incidence of breast cancer in women receiving estrogens for prolonged periods of time. (I know of no statistically valid evidence that the intermittent administration of progestins will diminish the incidence of breast cancer in women receiving estrogens.)

If the physician accepts these basic precepts of the "Feminine

Forever" program, he must also assume that (1) *many* premenopausal women and *all* postmenopausal women are estrogen-
deficient; (2) that administration of estrogens and progestins to
premenopausal women who are still actively menstruating will
retard specific aging processes; and (3) that prolonged estrogen,
that is, prolonged beyond the usual twenty-first-to-twenty-fifth-
day method of administration, is necessary to effect the desired
results.

Scientific evidence does not support these assumptions. During
the first year or so after cessation of menstruation, analysis of
estrogens in the urine or blood showed, in one study, that the
levels in these patients were not appreciably diminished from those
obtained during the normal menstrual cycle. Examination of the
cells of the vagina, the so-called "feminity index" during early
menopause, ages forty-five to sixty, has shown an excellent estrogen (or cornification) index in almost twenty-five per cent of
patients. Even during late menopause, ages sixty-one to eighty-
five, a high estrogen index has been found in 5 per cent of patients.
It would seem, therefore, that *all* patients are not deficient.

The "feminity index" has received wide publicity. It is done
in the doctor's office at the same time he does a "Pap" smear for
cervical cancer. Actually, the estrogen effect can be determined
on the same slide, but I prefer to do the index separately and read
it myself, since the Pap smear must be sent to a laboratory for
processing and the report is not available for forty-eight hours.
The technique is simple! A cotton-tipped applicator is drawn over
the side wall of the vagina to collect the surface cells, then dipped
in a test tube containing a salt solution. A special stain is added, and
one or two drops of this solution are examined under the microscope. Cells that have been stimulated by estrogen are square,
pink, have sharp edges and a very small nuclei. The cells at the
lowest level (basal cells) are round, polygonal, blue, and have a
large nucleus. These blue cells predominate when estrogen is lacking. In a matter of a minute, it is possible to tell rather accurately
whether the vagina is under the influence of adequate estrogen or
not. Unfortunately, the test may be spoiled by douching, by tampons, or by infections. Therefore, minute calculations are frequently worthless.

The "feminity index" has become a fetish with many women. Some even visit the office each month to have it performed. Sometimes this attitude even rubs off on the husband. The husband of one of my patients calls after each visit to ask for a precise determination of her estrogen-affected cells—much as he would call his broker for the latest Dow-Jones averages.

Not everyone is enthusiastic about the index. Experienced cytologists who read these vaginal smears have criticized the percentage of cornified cells stated to be desirable. They point out that the desired levels are much higher than those usually seen in women with normal menstrual cycles. Most gynecologists object strenuously to the recommendation that estrogen levels of the premenopausal women be increased and regular bleeding insured on the basis of an altered femininity index. They disagree with the notion of treating "primarily and principally the vaginal smear, not the symptoms."

Premenopausal women who have *regular, ovulatory* menstrual cycles have normal femininity indices in the vaginal smear and normal levels of estrogen in their blood. Unfortunately, many women in this age group have been misinformed. The impropriety of diagnosing "early menopause" in the presence of normal menstrual function is embarrassingly illustrated on occasion by the occurrence of pregnancy. Every so often, the "last egg in the basket" is released at age forty-eight or forty-nine. If fertilized, a most unwanted pregnancy results.

Therefore, I believe most emphatically that symptoms should not be ascribed to estrogen insufficiency on the basis of the patient's chronologic age. Some women have premature menopause because of ovarian infection or disease (endometriosis) during their late twenties or early thirties. Other women continue to ovulate regularly until age fifty or fifty-two. Certainly incipient menopause should not be diagnosed prior to the establishment of some degree of amenorrhea, scanty flow, or prolonged cycles.

It is important at this point to examine in detail a few misconceptions regarding the effects of estrogen-progestin.

1. *Hormones will restore youthful breasts.* Neither estrogen alone nor estrogen-progestin combinations or estrogen creams ap-

plied to the skin will restore breast tissue in aging women. Applied externally, the estrogen does nothing. Taken internally, the estrogen may maintain some engorgement of existing tissue and prevent sagging. But the best advice to an older woman who wishes a younger appearing bosom is to buy a good bra and hold herself up straight. Exercises that strengthen the muscles under the breasts may be helpful.

2. *The Pill will restore facial contour and texture.* This concept still awaits confirmation by controlled studies. I have seen women who have had their ovaries removed at an early age, and who were treated by constant estrogens, still develop skin wrinkling at the usual age. Conversely, other women who undergo menopause spontaneously at age forty have smooth, finely textured skin seven to ten years later without added estrogens. Obviously, this is an inherited trait similar to flowing hair or perfect teeth. Diet, general health, climate, and exercise are more a factor in skin condition than estrogen.

3. *The pills prevent or cure osteoporosis.* It is widely accepted that postmenopausal osteoporosis is an insidious process that often goes unsuspected until its presence is announced by pain induced by some trivial trauma, from a minor jolt in an automobile accident, to stepping down quickly from a high step. More than 1.5 million women in the United States have asymptomatic vertebral fractures, and over 10 million have lost 30 to 40 per cent of their vertebral bone and nearly as much compact bones in their hands as a result of this disease. These figures do not include the 3 to 4 million women estimated to have spinal osteoporosis. In its most serious form, the bones become porous, spongy, weakened. The spinal column tends to shorten, and the height diminishes as the "hump back" develops. The risk of falling increases and bones are broken easily. Since estrogen is necessary for the production of bone and connective tissue, a handful of physicians contend they can restore normal bone density in old people by giving them estrogens. However, the conservative *Medical Letter* summarizes current opinion among leading bone specialists and gynecologists as follows: "Restoration of normal bone density in postmenopausal osteoporosis has never been achieved by any measures." We still do not have

sufficient data to state that estrogen or the estrogen-progestin pill will *prevent* the development of osteoporosis. Even young women (and men) develop osteoporosis in certain bones when a limb is placed in a cast after a fracture—even in the presence of normal hormonal levels. The most that may be said at this time, I believe, is that while estrogen will not *cure* osteoporosis, it may cause marked improvement in the symptoms of the disease and retard its progression.* More exercise and activity, plus a proper diet with more milk, are important in preventing osteoporosis.

4. *Estrogens administered to the pre- and postmenopausal female will protect against premature development of heart disease.* Around 1850, the average life span of women was only two or three years more than of men. This statistical difference has slowly widened, and the expanding gap is now considerable, leaving about 10 million widows in the United States today. The burning question of the moment is why women live longer. Does the estrogen in their blood vessels really prevent the development of hardening of the arteries, particularly in the coronary vessels of the heart? Or is it related to less stress and worry? Or possibly to the fact that they smoke less? Is it because of hyper-hormonal states of pregnancy? There is no doubt that one factor is the diminished incidence of coronary artery disease in women during the third and fourth decades of life.

One of the most interesting features about coronary heart disease is the different incidence in men and women. Men in their thirties and forties develop the disease much more frequently than women, but in their fifties, the gap narrows, and after sixty the rate becomes almost equal. This has brought about much of the speculation as to why women are so much more protected against coronary heart disease. Since the estrogen production diminished at the same time that the increased incidence of coronary heart

* A recent report concerns the therapeutic effect of a new hormone, thyrocalcitonin, which is produced by the thyroid gland. Synthesized by Sandoz, Lederle, and Ciba, the hormone has been effective in treating osteoporosis and other bone diseases, as well as breast cancer, which often spreads to bones. Thyrocalcitonin is not commercially available and is classified as an experimental drug. Its side effects are unknown so far.

disease occurred, a natural but unscientific conclusion would be that the increased heart disease was due to diminished estrogen.

There is no scientific evidence at present to support the contention that women on estrogen-replacement therapy will have "protection" against heart disease. What is needed are large, randomized, controlled studies of treated vs. untreated postmenopausal women with regard to subsequent development of coronary artery disease. Laboratory studies and animal investigations do indicate the efficacy of treatment with estrogen. Since estrogen diminishes cholesterol and does produce improvement in EKG (electrocardiogram) changes in both men and women *with* coronary heart diseases, treatment of female patients is advised. This is definitive therapy, not prevention.

The best that can be said about estrogen therapy and heart disease are these words: *don't know*. In one recent report there was no clear evidence that diminished ovarian function per se made a woman more vulnerable to coronary disease. Apparently the higher coronary death rate in older women "approaches" the male rate not because of some sudden loss of protection, but rather because of a decreased male death rate, probably due to loss of large numbers of relatively young, male heart-attack victims. There is also no doubt that cultural, racial, and economic factors may also play a role, since the American Negro female is almost as susceptible to heart disease as the male.

USES OF ESTROGEN THERAPY

Treatment with hormones will seldom, if ever, live up to the claims of its proponents; nevertheless, the hormones are extremely useful to the physician seeking to treat a variety of disorders associated with menopause. Whether these disorders constitute a disease is a question of semantics. However, Dr. Allan C. Barnes, Professor of Obstetrics and Gynecology at Johns Hopkins University School of Medicine, has suggested that, because of its ravaging effects on the body, menopause should be considered a disease and treated as such. The only argument in favor of considering the condition a "natural" one was, in his mind, that menopause happened to all women. However, he pointed out that neglecting menopause medically simply because it is universal is unsound reasoning. "Death is also universal, yet we struggle against it," he said.

Estrogen is extremely valuable for the following purposes in the management of the menopausal woman:

1. Estrogen may be used to relieve the vaso-motor symptoms of menopause, including hot flashes, flushes, sweats, and insomnia. These occur in about 15 per cent of the patients.

2. Estrogen, either orally or by local application of creams, is extremely beneficial to the patient experiencing changes in her vagina that result in painful intercourse. Taken orally, estrogen frequently relieves some difficulties of urination.

3. Estrogen is definitely indicated in patients below the age of fifty following surgical removal of the ovaries or in patients born without ovaries.

4. Estrogen is useful in osteoporosis and in women with overt evidence of clinical coronary heart disease, as well as those women known to be predisposed to coronary artery disease. The latter group includes patients with high blood pressure, obesity, diabetes, or a familial disease known as hypercholesterolemia (high blood cholesterol levels).

Notably absent from this list of indications for estrogen therapy are such "cosmetic" purposes as improving breasts, beautifying complexion, and keeping a woman young. Is there nothing to be said for the "Feminine Forever" school of therapy? If a particular meaning is applied to the term "feminine forever," then I believe estrogen therapy has a specific effect. If remaining feminine implies absence of hot flashes and other vaso-motor symptoms; preservation of a normal and functional vagina; improved vigor and better health due to maintenance of normal protein metabolism; and less concern about the ravage of bone and heart disease, then I heartily agree with the advocates of femininity *ad infinitum*. But too many women have either been deluded or have a misconception concerning the basic problem. To them, the phrase "feminine forever" is synonymous with not growing old. They have the erroneous and quite sad notion that their skin won't age, that their breasts will remain young and firm, and that they, somehow, will achieve what Ponce de Leon sought in vain.

HAZARDS OF ESTROGEN THERAPY

If estrogen can bring benefits to the postmenopausal woman, there are also hazards associated with use of this hormone. The major difficulties concern the uterus and breasts and are due to restimulation of organs which, in menopause, have become quiescent. Fibroids may grow suddenly and produce intermittent staining or profuse bleeding. Sudden enlargement may produce symptoms from pressure of the fibroid on the bladder or rectum. If estrogens and progestins are given in sequence, endometriosis may be reactivated.

If an excessive amount of estrogen is given to a postmenopausal patient, bleeding will occur. This is not true menstruation since, by definition, menstruation follows ovulation, and these women do not ovulate. The postmenopausal woman is barren. If bleeding occurs after menopause, it must be accepted as a cancer "alarm," since in about half the patients who bleed during the postmenopause, cancer of the female genital tract is found. Unfortunately, there is only one certain way to make an accurate diagnosis and that is by D. and C. It would be a fatal error on the part of the patient, or the physician, to assume that the bleeding was *due* to the estrogen overdosage, since a cancer of the endometrium might have developed during the period of therapy.

As I will describe in the section on treatment of the postmenopausal female, estrogen is administered in the lowest possible dose, but in amounts adequate to relieve signs and symptoms of insufficiency *without* producing bleeding. Occasionally a patient may wish to bleed cyclically after menopause for psychological reasons. I recall a patient, an actress, who requested that I permit her to have withdrawal bleeding because she was married to a somewhat younger man and wished to maintain a monthly proof of youth. But most women, having endured menstruation for forty years or more, are quite grateful when it mercifully ends.

But there is greater danger with estrogen therapy than simply producing withdrawal bleeding. While there is no evidence that short courses of estrogen, properly prescribed and supervised, will *cause* cancer of the uterus, cellular growth may be stimulated.

Excessive or prolonged doses of estrogen may produce hyperplasia or overgrowth of the endometrium. The more florid type of overgrowth has a potential of malignancy of about 10 per cent.

There seems to be no evidence that estrogen *causes* breast cancer. However, the hormones are not to be used, according to regulation of the U. S. Food and Drug Administration, when there is presence or history of breast or genital cancer in the patient.

Perhaps the greatest danger of estrogen therapy is that the patient, lured by the promise of restored youth, will look in the mirror and decide to speed the clock on its backward movement by taking more pills than her physician prescribed. Or, when told to go off estrogen from time to time, she may decide instead to keep on taking them, an excellent way to produce hyperplasia. Or, she may neglect to return to the doctor for her required checkup. Or, she may bleed without telling her doctor. In all such cases, she is inviting serious difficulties that, put quite bluntly, may keep her feminine not at all.

There are other contraindications to the use of estrogen. These include women with serious liver disease, e.g. cirrhosis; some rare vascular diseases that predispose the patient to widespread blood clotting and heart failure; and large fibroid tumors of the uterus. Also, many women cannot tolerate estrogen because of distressing side effects, such as nausea, weight gain, and breast tenderness.

In spite of the risks of estrogen-replacement therapy, hormone pills are unquestionably here to stay. Their effectiveness in many conditions has been proved and is accepted by millions of persons, but they must be treated with respect. Physicians are, by and large, prescribing them judiciously. When, at a recent meeting of obstetricians and gynecologists, 2,200 doctors were asked if they prescribed estrogens, about 90 per cent said, "Yes, when needed."

TREATMENT OF THE PREMENOPAUSAL FEMALE

Women have an inordinate fear of menopause. Many women, as they reach their late forties, begin to observe symptoms of menopause, or what they believe to be symptoms, and panic. A woman in premenopause looks at her husband. He may be a year or two

older, but he is still active and virile. He is at the peak of his earn-
ing power. As she looks at him, she wonders how to keep from
losing him to a younger, more attractive woman. Unfortunately,
menopause comes at a difficult time in marriage. The couple has
been married twenty or twenty-five years, and their children are
married or away at college. The cement of family life comes un-
stuck, and the couple is asked to rediscover a marital relationship
they had when they were first wed. But now familiarity may have
bred contempt and, even worse, boredom. As the popular saying
goes, the "honeymoon has been over" for some time.

In my practice, patients frequently ask for estrogen therapy
years before they need it. They've read about the youth-restoring
properties of hormones, and they hope that pills will restore the
lost affection in their marriage. Many patients describe the symptoms of premenstrual tension, but believe they are caused by premature menopause. They are not estrogen-deficient; they have
an excess of sex hormones. I've had other patients ask for estrogen
because they have drooping breasts, flabby musculature, and facial
skin dryness with excessive wrinkling. These women are still in
their early forties, ovulating and menstruating normally. They are
not deficient in estrogen. They have symptoms of *hormonal imbalance,* perhaps even relative excesses of either estrogen or progesterone. The physical signs of aging are the result of heredity, poor
diet, lack of exercise, worry, stress or just overwork and inadequate
periods of rest and relaxation. I am constantly amazed at the
appearance of increased age of patients that I see in the clinic, compared to those in private practice. Although I do not see male
patients, I have been assured by my urologist friends that the same
is true in large wards of city hospitals. The overworked, financially
destitute, poorly nourished male of forty-five may appear to be
fifty-five or sixty. Money may not buy health, but extreme lack of it
may be responsible for illness and disease.

The first step in management of the premenopausal patient is
psychotherapy. I don't suggest that the services of a psychiatrist or
clinical psychologist are required, but the patient needs a sympathetic "hearing." The physiology of menopause should be explained, and the patient should be told which symptoms are due

to estrogen insufficiency and which are not. She needs to realize that menopause is not the end of life, but the beginning of a new one. New freedoms should be enjoyed, activities in the home and community extended, dormant interests reactivated, and unfulfilled ambitions renewed with vigor. The last thing she needs is a prescription by a physician, or, even worse, his nurse, for a "shotgun" preparation containing mixtures of hormone, sedative, stimulant, tranquilizer, and vitamins. Instead, the interested physician will help her face an elemental and interesting life process by dispelling fantasies, dissipating phobias, and correcting misconceptions.

The second step in treatment is to offer *specific* therapy for correction of *specific* symptoms. It must be emphasized that perhaps 85 per cent of all women pass through menopause easily, almost blithely, without noting any abnormality. Fine! I tell these patients to have a good time, relax, and forget about themselves. I suggest an examination and Pap smear once a year and caution them to return if irregular, profuse, or abnormal bleeding occurs. Minor complaints such as constipation and indigestion may be corrected by increased fluid intake, regular exercise, and improvement in dietary habits. A few patients may need a tranquilizer or mild sedative to assist them through temporary periods of stress or anxiety. Another distressing symptom complex, premenstrual tension, has been discussed in Chapter 16, but it may occur frequently in the premenopausal patient. Relief may be obtained by explanation, a low salt diet, diuretics, and mild sedatives. But one thing is eminently clear: the patients with normal menstrual cycles do *not* need estrogen replacement therapy.

If the patient has hot and cold flashes, insomnia, painful intercourse, and skips and delays of periods, she has entered a later phase of premenopause, and her symptoms are specifically due to estrogen insufficiency. In my experience, reassurance, tranquilizers, mood elevators, and diuretics are now inadequate. To accomplish optimum improvement, the hormonal deficiency must be corrected. This brings us to the third step in the management of menopause, the use of sex hormones, estrogen and progesterone.

The hormonal management of such patients involves the use of estrogen-progestin agents in the exact dosage and regimen of the Pill. The sequential oral contraceptives are particularly advantageous for the premenopausal patient, for they more nearly duplicate the natural hormonal cycle. The sequential pills, such as Oracon and C-Quens, have been discussed previously. Also useful in managing the premenopausal patient is Profem (Upjohn).* It is an "everyday" pill in which the patient receives .025 mg. of estrogen for seven days, .1 mg. of estrogen for the next fourteen days, then .125 mg. of estrogen plus progestin for the remaining seven days of the cycle. When the patient returns to the beginning of the regimen, menstruation occurs. Profem has the advantage of providing the premenopausal patient with a small amount of estrogen during the time she is menstruating. But all sequential agents have the advantage of affording relief from the symptoms of estrogen insufficiency, while protecting the patient from pregnancy.

Certain patients will note excessive withdrawal bleeding while taking the sequential agents. This is particularly true of patients who have histories of excessive flow. If "withdrawal" or "breakthrough" bleeding is recurrent, a curettage should be done to exclude the possibility of an organic cause. Subsequent treatment should be with a combination pill such as Norinyl-2, Ortho-Novum-2, or Ovulen. These are taken in twenty- or twenty-one-day cycles, exactly the same as the Pill used for contraceptive purposes.

Treatment of the premenopausal patient is continued until the average age of menopause, about fifty to fifty-two years. This is not absolute, however, and if patients request that cyclic withdrawal bleeding be discontinued at age forty-eight or forty-nine, they are then placed on the regimens of estrogen therapy, if indicated. Similarly, certain patients appear younger, both mentally and physically, than their chronological age. If they desire to remain on premenopausal therapy until age fifty-four or fifty-five, I see no reason for not doing so.

Abnormal bleeding, of any type, during the administration of estrogen-progestin sequential or combination agents should be

---

* Profem has been investigated in clinical trials for over two years but has not, as yet, been marketed.

investigated with the same thoroughness as abnormal bleeding in patients of this age group who are not receiving therapy. For minimal breakthrough bleeding, an endometrial biopsy and endometrial aspiration for cytology is usually adequate. Pap smears are done annually, and examination of the genital organs and breasts is done every six months. A thorough uterine curettage must be done in all patients having recurrent breakthrough or heavy withdrawal bleeding. An organic cause is usually found. Patients with previous endometrial hyperplasia who are being treated by cyclic estrogen-progestin therapy should have a curettage every six months until the hyperplasia has disappeared. This sounds like an excessive number of surgical procedures necessitating hospital admissions. Actually, however, I have observed almost two hundred patients in this group and have never found recurrence of the hyperplasia *as long as the estrogen-progestin combination was continued.* Progestins and hyperplasia of the endometrium are not compatible bedfellows and I have not seen a recurrence of this process, nor its initiation during treatment. This is not to say, however, that once the Pill has been discontinued, hyperplasia will not return. This depends on the ability of the ovary to secrete estrogen after cessation of medication. For this reason many gynecologists elect to perform a vaginal hysterectomy, especially if other reasons exist.

TREATMENT OF THE POSTMENOPAUSAL FEMALE

Treatment of the woman who has entered the postmenopausal period of life differs from that of the premenopausal female in two ways: (1) ovulation need not be suppressed for conception control; and (2) regular withdrawal bleeding is not necessary. Such bleeding is a nuisance and has been given undue importance as a factor in the prevention of breast and uterine cancer.

Approximately 30 per cent of women will have had menopause, that is, one full year without a menstrual period, by age forty-five; 60 per cent by age fifty; 98 per cent by age fifty-five; and 100 per cent by the age of sixty. In a woman with evidence of estrogen insufficiency, the administration of estrogen may be a Godsend;

but this hormone must be given with meticulous care. No two patients are exactly the same, neither in their appearance nor in their response to medications, especially hormonal agents. For a physician (or his nurse) to hand out pills or prescriptions on an assembly-line basis is to be abhorred. Every patient must be carefully observed and her symptoms recorded to be certain that the proper amount of estrogen is being administered.

I have advised treatment of the postmenopausal female for the following indications: (1) vasomotor symptoms such as hot flashes, flushes, sweats; (2) insomnia without cause; (3) atrophy (thinning) of the vaginal and bladder lining, especially if there is painful intercourse; (4) bilateral removal of the ovaries for diseases other than cancer of the uterus or breast; (5) osteoporosis; (6) coronary artery disease or those conditions that predispose to coronary artery disease in the female (hypercholesterolemia, which means excessive blood cholesterol, diabetes, excessive cigarette smoking, obesity, hypertension, thyroid disease).

If the uterus has not been removed, I prescribe an oral estrogen, to be taken at bedtime from the first to the twenty-first day of each month. If nausea is bothersome, the pill should be taken with the evening meal. There are several estrogens on the market, and some are better tolerated than others. A patient may have nausea with one but not another. Swelling and weight gain may be troublesome to patients who ingest, unknown to themselves, large amounts of salt.

The most commonly used estrogenic substances are: Premarin (sodium estrone sulfate), Estinyl (ethinyl estradiol), diethylstilbestrol (DES), Vallestril, and Tace. If hot flashes and sweats do not disappear in a week or ten days, I instruct the patient to double the dose during the next cycle. If these symptoms are bothersome during the nine or ten days during which estrogen is not being taken, I suggest a twenty-five-day schedule each month. But under no circumstances do I prescribe estrogens constantly, if the uterus is present. The risks of hyperplasia of the endometrium are too great, even if the dose of estrogen is small. Some physicians do prescribe constant estrogen, without the use of a progestin to produce "withdrawal flowing," but to avoid breakthrough bleeding and hyperplasia, a very low dose must be given. In my opinion, this dose is inadequate to produce the optimum effects in this treatment program.

Frequently, the nipples will become tingly and the breasts full and tender. These symptoms usually indicate an excess of estrogen with resultant fluid retention in breast tissues. It occurs more frequently in women who are taking estrogen constantly. If the uterus has been removed for a nonmalignant condition, one need not worry about bleeding or hyperplasia. Therefore, I usually give estrogen daily to these patients. However, if the breast symptoms noted above occur, I again utilize the twenty-one- to twenty-five-day cycles of treatment. In addition, the breast tenderness may be diminished by the following methods: use of a diuretic agent for three or four days; a low salt diet; reduction in the amount of daily estrogen; addition of male hormone (testosterone) to the prescription because of its anti-estrogenic effect.

In my opinion, the only woman who should receive estrogen daily is the patient who has had her uterus removed, since in these patients there is no risk of hyperplasia. In fact, the treatment of estrogen insufficiency is greatly simplified if the patient no longer has a uterus. Dr. M. Edward Davis, with tongue in cheek, has suggested a radical approach—"Take out everyone's uterus after age 40, then give as much estrogen as needed." Although this sounds drastic, I have treated several patients who, even on small doses of estrogen, developed recurrent bleeding from fibroid tumors in the lining of the uterus. After trying several treatment schemes, it became obvious that estrogen could not be given. These patients elected to have a hysterectomy, then take their estrogens. None have been sorry they made this decision.

At present, no treatment schedule can guarantee the absence of estrogen-induced bleeding if the woman still has her uterus. However, small doses are less likely to cause uterine bleeding and to produce annoying side effects. Therefore, the smallest dose should be given first, then increased on the basis of persistent symptoms. One must be careful, however, not to assume that all hot flashes, sweats, and insomnia are due to estrogen insufficiency. Thyroid disease, particularly hyperthyroidism, hypertension, or other diseases of the small blood vessels may produce similar symptoms.

I caution my patients carefully about bleeding. A small amount of staining or scanty flow is permitted as a "withdrawal" effect. This is a result of the growth of the endometrium when estrogen is taken and its degeneration during the period of off-treatment. If this is recurrent or profuse, I do a biopsy or Pap smear. Curettage of the uterus is indicated if either of these tests is abnormal.

Bleeding should never occur during the days estrogen is taken. This is called breakthrough bleeding and usually signifies some abnormality within the uterus. It may be a polyp, a fibroid, or hyperplasia. In any event, a curettage must always be performed.

Recent medical literature has cited evidence that very early cancer of the endometrium may be stimulated to bleed by estrogens before any other symptoms are noted. For example, I have several patients who were placed on estrogens because of hot flashes and sweats. Although these patients had not had bleeding during the three or four years since menopause, they noted intermittent spotting within six to eight weeks. A curettage revealed very early cancer, and hysterectomies were performed. These women were lucky! They were cured simply because a very early diagnosis was possible. Unfortunately, the Pap smear, intrauterine aspirations, and even an endometrial biopsy will not always detect cancer of the endometrium in its earliest state.

I do not administer injectable estrogens for the relief of hot flashes, sweats, and other symptoms when the uterus is present. The length of the action is unpredictable, and the cumulative effect usually results in irregular bleeding from excessive growth of the uterine lining.

All oral estrogens have similar effects, and I have no preference for natural estrogens, except for their improved tolerance, that is, less nausea and gastrointestinal upsets. Premarin is a "natural" estrogen obtained from the urine of pregnant mares. It is actually "estrone," a metabolic product of the basic estrogen made in the human ovary, estradiol. The only difference is that estrone has one less atom of oxygen and hydrogen. The other estrogens marketed today are synthetics. The closest one to estradiol is Estinyl. Tace and Vallestril are similar to DES, the first estrogen synthesized.

DES is quite cheap, but has the greatest number of undesirable side effects. When given in low dosage, however, it is quite well tolerated.

Pharmaceutical companies are searching for the "ideal" estrogen. Such a compound would alleviate undesirable symptoms, retard degenerative changes in the bones and blood vessels, improve signs of hormonal insufficiency in the female genital tract, but would not overstimulate the lining of the uterus or the breasts. Clinical investigation is progressing favorably in this field, and the time is not too distant when newer agents will be available.

Many women, particularly those who are newly menopausal, continue to be troubled by anxiety-linked symptoms despite estrogen therapy. This is not unexpected since it is obvious that most psychic disturbances of the climacteric are *not* due to hormonal insufficiency. The depression of the climacteric period is probably the most common emotional finding. As in other forms of depression, there is usually an underlying degree of anger that is often related to loss of reproductive ability, as well as body image. When this is coupled with guilt feeling, the typical depression of the climacteric is noted.

The very narcissistic woman frequently is unable to tolerate the changes in her body image. She feels she has lost a considerable amount of sexual attractiveness and thinks no man finds her sexually interesting. She assiduously avoids sexual situations in which she feels she will be rejected. Such women go to extremes in purchases of worthless creams, ointments, teenage miniskirts, and even have major plastic surgery performed in the hope of restoring a youthful body image. These individuals are the first to run to their physician for a pill to restore their fading beauty.

Emotionally mature women realize that sexual attractiveness is much more than physical charm alone and are better able to accept changes in body image. Women who have had rewarding love experiences accept the physiological and anatomical changes of the menopausal years with greater dignity and calm than the spinster or the frigid woman. Women having this temperament and ability to adjust are frequently found to have fairly normal estrogen levels well beyond the time when their menstrual periods cease. For them, estrogen pills are unnecessary.

To summarize, estrogen is invaluable for the treatment of specific menopausal and postmenopausal symptoms, if given in the lowest possible dose and in a cyclical manner. There is no evidence that estrogen, so administered, will cause cancer of the uterus or breast. However, the Food and Drug Administration warns against the use of estrogens in the presence of or history of breast or genital cancer. The hormones must be given with caution to patients with liver disease, diabetes, fibroids, or heart disease.

Oral contraceptives are of exceptional value to the premenopausal woman who ovulates irregularly and has evidence of estrogen insufficiency.

The fountain of youth does not come in hormone pills. Nor does femininity. But, used with common sense, these pills can bring relief and comfort, safely and effectively, to the women who need them.

IV

PSYCHOLOGICAL, SOCIAL, AND MORAL EFFECTS OF THE PILL

19. The Pill and Your Mental Health

THE PHYSIOLOGICAL effects of the Pill, beneficial and detrimental, temporary and prolonged, rare and commonplace, are tangible matters to the gynecologist. His training and experience enable him to manage these complaints by manipulation of the medication and by other treatment. But emotional and psychosomatic complaints are not as easily solved.

A physician frequently finds it necessary to treat the mind as he heals the body. While his activity hardly rivals that of a psychiatrist or clinical psychologist, the physician, whether generalist or specialist, must counsel his patient in a way that permits complete understanding of the disease or disorder. The simple process of informing a patient about the nature of his or her illness, and its prognosis, frequently results in mental attitudes that aid specific therapy.

The Pill has generated a vast number of psychic as well as somatic (physical) complaints. I am certain that many of the somatic complaints originate via the cerebral cortex of the brain, and I suppose we should call these psychosomatic problems. The complaints include practically all of the symptoms listed in an excellent medical-student textbook called *Signs and Symptoms.* This is rather remarkable considering that the Pill has been marketed for less than a decade. Of the myriad symptoms noted, *fear* is foremost. At least fear is the initiating process, and a subsequent chain reaction involving many body systems follows. To illustrate: When I administer one of the newer chemotherapy drugs, such as methotrexate or cytoxan, to a patient with far-advanced cancer, I am seriously concerned about the side effects. I worry. I hope the drug will have its desirable effect on tumor cells without injuring normal ones. But the patient is not afraid, since the relief of symptoms and possible cure more than outweigh the disadvantage of serious side effects. I suppose it is not fair to compare a cancer patient taking a very toxic drug with a normal female taking one with minimal toxicity, but it really is a game of comparison of risk.

The point I would like to make is this: When a physician prescribes the Pill now, in 1969, any previous exposure of the patient to rumor-mongering or scare publicity immediately ignites smoldering worries and fears about cancer, blood clots, blindness, baldness and even death. I frequently try to put myself in the patient's place and ask myself if I would take the Pill if I knew as little about it as she does. But, despite the scares, the inaccuracies, the reports of isolated cases of this, that, and everything, most patients respect the judgment of their physicians. I do not agree with the writers of a recent *Ladies' Home Journal* article who implied that patients "forced" their physicians to give them the Pill. Nor do I believe that the opposite of this is true. Several recent studies have indicated that if a patient is given the facts honestly and fairly, she will select the best method of conception control for her purposes. Negating fear with precise information is a major task confronting every physician who prescribes the Pill or inserts an intrauterine device.

The variety of psychological complaints associated with the Pill require much more than simple information to effect adequate treatment. Such complaints seem more suitable for a psychotherapist, a marriage counselor, a clergyman, a sociologist, or even a philosopher. The physician must blend a bit of each of these professions into his own. But, even accomplishing this, his problem is compounded by the extreme variety of complaints. Whereas one patient may exclaim, "I feel positively euphoric when I take the Pill," another may complain, as did the mother of three children, "I just sat there in the morning with the house falling down around me. I'd cry over nothing. I couldn't face the day."[26] (I've heard the same complaint from women not taking the Pill soon after they find themselves pregnant for the fourth or fifth time.) Still another patient comments, "It alters my whole attitude toward sex. I feel completely relaxed now." Hardly justifiable as a complaint, you might say. True, but the very next patient may sadly state, "I feel pregnant all the time. I don't want to make love. I just want to go to sleep."[26] Not quite as bad, but still worrisome, is this complaint, "I have a sort of apathy, a dampening of enthusiasm, both physical and emotional, that just does not seem to go away."

A recent study by Dr. Ruth Lidz, Associate Professor of Clinical Psychiatry at Yale University, offers an explanation for many of these reactions. Dr. Lidz suggests that it may be the extreme efficacy of the Pill, rather than its chemical action, that leads to depression in some women. Her study of emotional reactions to contraception indicated that "Whenever the contraceptive, however rationally indicated and even wanted by the woman, counters a strong emotional need or undermines a neurotic adjustment, we may find reactions of frustration, depression, guilt, and frequently marital difficulties." Dr. Lidz suggests that a less-effective birth control method "that allows for more fantasy of perhaps getting pregnant" may be more psychologically acceptable to many women, especially those who lack strong motivation for fertility control.

There are other sources for psychosomatic display of underlying mental conflict. Many women fear that their "new freedom" may lead to promiscuity, particularly if this latent desire has been held in abeyance by fear of pregnancy. Catholic women may have guilt feelings about using the Pill, even if sanctioned by their parish priest, since approval has been denied by the Vatican. The reaction of the husband has received scant attention, but, as described in the next chapter, his appraisal and attitude may lead to difficult marital problems.

There is another problem of even greater magnitude. As we continue to develop improved and longer-acting methods of contraception, additional moral and philosophical issues will arise. For example, a postintercourse approach to contraception, the so-called "morning after" pill, is now being evaluated in several research centers. Its use poses two major questions: (1) would such a pill encourage promiscuity and further the deterioration of society's traditional attitude toward chastity? and (2) would such a pill be an abortifacient? The latter question involves the thorny problem of when life begins. In addition, there are demographic issues concerning the threat of over-population and theological controversies such as the attitude of the Catholic Church toward conception control.

These are not specific *medical* problems in the usual sense of the word, but the medical profession is intimately involved. Since physicians and scientists developed the Pill and are now engaged in testing newer methods, they must accept the responsibility of the effects produced in every parameter. Physicians prescribe oral contraceptives as a medication. They cannot, therefore, disclaim involvement in the psychological, moral, and social problems that ensue. Therefore it is appropriate to discuss these matters in this book.

DEPRESSION

The survey of physicians conducted by the American College of Obstetricians and Gynecologists, referred to so often because it represents the opinion of physicians dealing primarily with women, showed that emotional problems are more common among users of the Pill than was hitherto thought. Two out of five doctors attributed "personality change" to *some* patients taking the Pill. A few patients said the change was for the better, but most patients apparently thought the change was for the worse.

One of the forms of personality change most disturbing to patients is that of depression. Forty-one per cent of the ACOG members ranked depression among the five most frequent reasons for abandoning the Pill.

The first question to ask is whether the Pill really *causes* depression or simply unmasks an underlying, suppressed tendency. Unfortunately, this condition is universal, although it is not constant. Everyone has at least occasional "blue days" or bouts of depression. There are many causes: disappointments, frustration, "bad news," poor health, lack of rest, guilt about neglecting responsibilities, even the weather.

Is there something about the hormones in the Pill that causes depression? Evidence that estrogen and progesterone, natural body hormones, cause depression is scanty and unconvincing. Some physicians believe that a state of depression may be related to bloating caused by salt and water retention. They hypothesize that increased fluid in brain tissues depresses the central nervous system. However, autopsies on women killed accidentally and who were using the Pill have not verified this theory. Other physicians have suggested that the progestin in the Pill may be soporific (sleep inducing). There is no doubt that progesterone, if given to animals in large doses, can actually induce sleep to the point where surgery may be performed. The latest estrogen-progestin compounds have extremely small amounts of hormones per tablet. Yet even these mini-doses may depress overly sensitive individuals. The majority of Pill users are not bothered by this side effect and a few actually take advantage of it. A young woman who has been taking the Pill since 1958 explains, "I found that initially I had trouble because I was very tired; but the pill was then being given in ten-milligram doses and furthermore I was taking it in the morning. Now I take a pill containing only 5 mg. in the evening. I think it helps me sleep."[38]

A few women complain of "a sort of apathy, a lack of functioning; an inability to really move; a kind of heaviness, both physical and emotional; no vitality; a dampening of enthusiasm that just doesn't seem to go away.[38] When I review the history of such a patient, I frequently find that excessive energy was never part of her makeup. As a matter of fact, quite a few have been downright lazy. For patients exhibiting this response, I obtain four tests to exclude organic disease. These are: a chest x-ray to rule out tuberculosis; a red-blood cell count and hematocrit to be certain that anemia is not present; a blood glucose to exclude diabetes; and thyroid function tests. About one in twenty patients will show some abnormality. The rest are just plain overworked, either physically or emotionally, or both. Some are tired of their "situation," tired of their job, their home life, their husband, the humdrum monotony of day-to-day life. An amazing recovery occurs, even while taking the Pill, if a vacation from the "tiring milieu" is possible.

Clinical investigators and psychiatrists doubt that the Pill causes depression because of a specific hormonal effect on the nervous system. After all, the Pill contains hormones very similar to those produced by the ovary each month. Furthermore, the amount of hormone, particularly in the newer pills, approximates the amount produced at the time of ovulation. Depressed states are not commonly associated with ovulation, nor are they a frequent finding after ovulation when the estrogen-progesterone levels are highest. As a matter of record, most depressions occur just prior to menstruation when the levels of estrogen and progesterone are at low ebb!

Yet, a certain number of Pill users do complain of depressed states. Dr. Selig Neubardt, an obstetrician-gynecologist, has noted that such depression occurs very subtly, frequently not starting until seven or eight months have passed, much beyond the time when the other side effects have disappeared.[39] The depression may be aggravated each subsequent month, but most women do not recognize it as being pill related. There are instances of dramatic cure, both with and without psychiatric consultation, by simply discontinuing the Pill.

It is difficult to determine the exact incidence of depression in users of oral contraceptives. Dr. Neubardt estimates that 1 to 2 per cent of his patients became so depressed while taking the Pill that they gave it up.[39] On the other hand, Sam Blum, writing in *Redbook*, quotes the director of a clinical study in a large Boston hospital, "We were particularly looking for depression and just not finding much of it. The results of interviews and standard psychological testing showed that the pills did not appear to affect the group's depression score in any way, although a number of individual women reacted, some for better, some for worse."³⁸

Until a specific physiological correlation between the Pill and depression is demonstrated, this complaint must be considered as an emotional or psychosomatic response. Yet it is virtually impossible to predict which patients will develop depression. One might expect that a past history of nervous or mental disease would be a predisposing factor. Occasionally it is, but usually the patient noting depression has a negative past history and has done extremely well on the Pill. Furthermore, she usually has had fewer side effects than other patients.

While psychiatrists and clinical investigators are not likely to accept a direct effect of the Pill on the cerebral cortex as a cause of depression, most will agree that the mere physical act of Pill taking may evoke this response. One physician commented, "It would be amazing if there were no reactions. Women have idiosyncracies. Anything might depress them. Any drug, including sugar pills or aspirin, taken regularly, can lead to depression. The Pill is being taken by a lot of women who have serious psychological problems about contraception and sex. Those problems can come out in side reactions, depressions—who knows what else?"³⁸

Depression is a common reaction to disappointment and frustration. In reviewing the survey of the ACOG, Alice Lake noted that some women wove fantasies about the benefits of the Pill and became disappointed when it failed to live up to their dreams.²⁶ One of the more popular misconceptions is that the Pill, by relieving the fear of pregnancy, will change a woman from a reluctant or passive sexual partner into an aggressive, passionate one. Often this is exactly what happens. "It alters your whole attitude toward sex," says a 37-year-old mother quoted in *McCall's*.²⁶ "I feel completely relaxed now. Before, there was always the thought of an accident in the back of my mind." Unfortunately, however, not all users react in this way. Two young Catholic women interviewed by Blum had precisely opposite responses to the Pill.³⁸ One who had been "preoccupied with pregnancy" was unable to secure sexual gratification from intercourse. But after starting the Pill she enjoyed complete sexual harmony. Obviously an improvement in her "level of depression" followed. The other, "a tense and immature woman," was a prime example of one having "pregnancy phobia" and unfortunately she equated this phobia with fear of the act of intercourse. She lost her fear of pregnancy after beginning oral contraceptives, but sexual satisfaction was not forthcoming. Of course she was disappointed! This patient simply expected too much from the Pill; she hoped that conception control and sexual gratification would be intimately wrapped up in a neat little package. Needless to say, her "depression rating" dipped to a new low. But perhaps this effect of the Pill is salutary. At least it brought into the open a basic, but correctible, psychosomatic conflict. Now she knew beyond all doubt that her fear was sex and the sex act—not the pregnancy which might have resulted. Thus the Pill takes on the property of unmasking hidden defects, mental, physical, and physiological. The prediabetic female may be forced to divulge her inability to metabolize sugar after using the Pill. But who is to say that this is detrimental? Knowing this a bit earlier in life might lead to improved planning—in diet, in weight gain, and in child spacing.

Psychiatrist Shepard Ginandes is quoted in *Redbook* as stating, "Most women with sex problems would much rather believe that they're afraid of pregnancy than admit that they hate sex, or have a moral or emotional hangup of some sort. In their society they know they're supposed to enjoy sex. After all, women enjoy it in Henry Miller and in Italian films and in *Playboy*, so if a woman doesn't, she's got to have reasons. Obviously it's better for her to say that she's afraid of something. She doesn't want to tell herself that she'd just rather not—tonight, or ever. The Pills take away her excuse for not really looking at her own feelings."[38]

Disappointment and subsequent depression may occasionally be the result of misleading articles that attribute an aphrodisiac quality to the Pill. I know of patients whose tubes were previously tied who tried the Pill for this quality alone. It was not successful.

There is no doubt that the Pill has aided and abetted the physical quality of intercourse among couples who consider mechanical devices unpleasant. But the Pill cannot create love where love does not exist nor improve intercourse between incompatible mates. Disappointment is inevitable when a woman (or her husband) expects the Pill to accomplish more than it was designed to do.

Another interesting psychological correlation between the Pill and depression has been noted in women who express the desire to use a contraceptive, but subconsciously wish to be pregnant. There is a relation between such ambivalence and depression. Women could maintain their devil-may-care ambivalence with the diaphragm, foams, or with rhythm. It was sort of an "ovulation roulette." If nothing happened, well fine! But if pregnancy occurred—OK, we'll take that too. Sam Blum, writing in *Redbook*,[38] has cited the example of a young college graduate who was extremely loving and the proud mother of three children. She explained with a smile that "Every last one of them was an accident. Two were the result of coming home from cocktail parties feeling lazy, lucky, and romantic, but the middle one—I just don't know what happened." This patient was glad about every accident, but now desires no more children and is taking the Pill. Although she has never noted a side effect, she is a good example of what Dr. E. James Lieberman of the National Institute of Mental Health means by stating that "With the old methods [of contraception] there was scope for the play of human ambivalence."

If a couple both do and do not want more children, they tend to play hit and miss in their contraceptive practice, says Dr. Lieberman, who continues, "Now, when you give a woman a foolproof method, this kind of flexibility doesn't exist and from the psychological point of view, we have reason to believe that if a person cannot have the necessary leeway for his unconscious conflicts to be worked out, the anxiety will have to be discharged in some other way."

Many of the women interviewed by Mr. Blum are perfectly aware of their ambivalence toward pregnancy. One patient asked, "Is any woman ever sure she wants no more babies?" Another commented, "Before the Pill, I was always worried about getting pregnant, but at the same time wishing I would. I have a strong desire to be pregnant. Before the Pill, I forgot the diaphragm quite a few times. I was always half hoping. But with the Pill I had to come to grips with the fact that I do not choose to be pregnant at this time, and so I did come to grips with it. There is plenty of time to be pregnant in the future."

Mr. Blum suggests that "By enabling a woman to separate sex from conception, the Pill brings her face-to-face not only with her true sexual nature, but also with her true maternal nature. The Pill, like so much else in current American life, requires women to make decisions and exercise choice, where in the past, necessity or tradition decided for them. It would be surprising if at least a few women did not become depressed when faced with reality and the choices it dictates." In this one paragraph I believe that Mr. Blum has successfully summarized one of the more serious side effects associated with use of the Pill.

LIBIDO

The major surprise of the ACOG questionnaire was the finding that 31 per cent of the doctors surveyed blamed the Pill for a reduction in the sex drive of their patients, while only 24 per cent reported that it increased the libido of patients. Other studies have achieved different results. In a planned-parenthood study, 32 per cent of the women reported an increase in libido. Some women lose interest in sex during pregnancy. These may be among the group who note less libido while taking the Pill.

Dr. Edris Rice-Wray has reported her findings based on interviews with seventy-four Pill users selected at random from thousands of poor and lower-middle-class Mexicans attending her clinic in Mexico City.[40] She reports, "Forty women stated that their sexual drive had increased, 30 said there was no change, while only four stated it was less. The group of 40 said that the frequency of sexual relations had also increased; two stated that sexual relations were less frequent than before." Dr. Rice-Wray also noted, "Those whose libido and frequency of sexual relations had increased attributed the change to the release from the constant fear of becoming pregnant again, a fear which had caused them so much anxiety and nervousness. One couple in this study had not had sexual relations for two years for fear of pregnancy."

Other investigators have also reported an increase in the frequency of sexual relations among the Pill-taking population. Dr. Ailon Shiloh, an Associate Professor of Anthropology at the University of Pittsburgh, studied the behavior of 239 women who applied to a local planned-parenthood center.[41] Eighty-five per cent of the women were married and between the ages of twenty and thirty-nine. About 10 per cent were age nineteen or younger.

Before birth control was started, the women were asked how they felt about sexual intercourse. Seventy per cent of the Catholics reported that they "enjoyed sex relations tremendously," as did 56 per cent of the white Protestants. Only 39 per cent of the Negroes had this reaction. Rather, 13 per cent of the Negro women found intercourse unpleasant, contrasted with 5 per cent of the white Protestants and 3 per cent of the white Catholics.

The women were also asked about the frequency of their sexual relations, again before taking the Pill. Both groups of white women had a higher frequency of intercourse than the Negroes, 22 per cent of the white women having sexual relations *four or more times a week*, compared to only 17 per cent of the Negroes. Before starting the Pill, the women were asked this question: "Do you feel the frequency of your sexual relations is too often, just about often enough, or not quite often enough?" Over 70 per cent indicated "just about often enough," 20 per cent said it was not often enough, and 9 per cent said it was too often.

After three months of Pill use, the same women were questioned again. The percentage of women finding sex unpleasant had dropped to 3 per cent in all groups. As to frequency of sex, those women who had reported having intercourse only once or twice a week reported having intercourse two or more times a week. The percentage of women who felt sex occurred too often declined from 9 per cent to 3 per cent. The percentage who felt their sexual relations occurred just about often enough went up to 82 per cent, while the percentage who felt they did not have intercourse often enough went down from 20 per cent to 15 per cent. Dr. Shiloh concluded by stating, "There are no pronounced changes as measured by the frequency of sex relations [in Pill users]. Doctors need not worry that their patients will become licentious if they advocate modern birth control technics such as the Pill. Rather they should bear in mind that women of all religions have sexual problems and that all seem to want the new technics. And once these are adopted, the women experience a greater enjoyment of sex."

Some decrease in the frequency of intercourse has been reported among patients using the new brands of Pills containing small doses of estrogen and progestin. This appears to result from a higher incidence of breakthrough bleeding, rather than diminished sex drive.

It is difficult to pinpoint a cause for any of the changes in libido or frequency of intercourse. The decrease in sexual desire may be caused by the feelings of pregnancy in the early cycles of Pill taking. Women experiencing excessive bloating or nausea understandably would be less amorous.

Certain physicians have offered a possible hormonal explanation for increased sex drive from the Pill. Psychiatrist Theodore Robie has said, "There is no doubt that progesterone, and in some cases estrogen, improves sexual responsiveness in some women who have minimal responses. It has been used in the treatment of frigidity." Dr. Robert Greenblatt, a noted endocrinologist, has given male hormone to his female patients who complain of frigidity, lack of libido, or inability to reach a climax. Greenblatt describes excellent results in a large percentage of patients. There is no doubt that male hormone increases the degree of congestion of the clitoris, and if the dose is excessive, it will actually enlarge, sometimes to the size of a small penis. If the manipulation of the base of the clitoris is as important for conjugal enjoyment in the sex act as some experts say, the use of male hormone can be easily explained. Since some of the progestins have certain androgenic (male) tendencies, increased libido while taking these agents is easily explained. Several of my patients have described this experience after changing from a female- to a male-type progestin. The observations are merely suggestive since other investigators doubt that estrogens or progestins have a direct effect on sex drive.

The empirical evidence derived from patients does not clarify the variation in sexual response. One patient told her gynecologist, "I had never known anything like it. It was as though I had never made love before. Now that I enjoy it, I want it every night." Some women report an increased sex drive—a few even to the point of nymphomania. But there are those who report a flattening of sexual interest with the Pill. "Something is wrong," a British woman told her doctor. "I've lost interest in sex."

An explanation for changes in libido seems to lie more in the realm of psychology than in physiology. One factor leading to increased enjoyment of sex must be the elimination of the mechanical unpleasantness and interruptions associated with diaphragms, condoms, and spermicidal jellies—no muss, no fuss! Closely related to this is the elimination of the fear of pregnancy. Thus, with the Pill, couples are able to enjoy uninterrupted foreplay and passion leading to a more natural form of intercourse, and yet be 100 per cent certain that an unwanted pregnancy will not result.

Obviously, such a form of intercourse is not an unmixed blessing. As previously noted, a woman who does not receive satisfaction from intercourse and has previously blamed this on fear of pregnancy or the unpleasantness of diaphragms or condoms may have to face the reality of her own lack of sexuality. In a social climate that emphasizes sexuality, the reality of her own frigidity may lead to a diminution of libido as an escape mechanism.

Excessive fear of cancer or blood clots may serve to dampen sexual urge, particularly if a recent article has emphasized these aspects of Pill use. Passion and sexual intercourse depend upon many psychological factors. A baby's cry, a sudden footstep, remembering she forgot to turn off the kitchen range or do the laundry can lead to a sudden loss of passion. Certainly, the woman who worries about the Pill affecting her health will have her sex desire diminished.

In the main, those women who have a satisfactory sexual relationship with their husbands do experience an increase in their sexual desire and frequency of intercourse because of the greater naturalness of the act and the alleviation of the fear of pregnancy. Women with an unsatisfactory relationship will find little in the Pill to improve it.

Thus far, the discussion has been entirely about the effect of the Pill on the wife. The Pill also has an interesting effect on some husbands, the subject of the next chapter.

20. The Pill and Your Husband

WHEN THE PILL first became available, it was thought that it would liberate the act of love from the spectre of pregnancy and that it would release pent-up womanly passion. Furthermore, it was assumed that all husbands would rejoice. Such liberation, reasoned many experts, would greatly enhance the quality of marital love. These assumptions, unfortunately, may not be universally true.

The theory underlying these basic ideas was that an improved sexual relationship would benefit all aspects of marriage. The early reports from gynecologists, psychologists, and sociologists forecast a reduction in marriage problems. After all the contraceptive was foolproof if used correctly. Inopportune delays for installation of a device were unnecessary. The moment of passion did not have to be placed on a strict time schedule. As one Catholic husband confided, "I'm sick of this S.O.S. [sex on schedule] routine. How can the church expect a couple to turn sex on and off like a light switch. Sexual relations should be guided by love, by emotion, by need and not by a schedule and not by one negative vote from Rome."

Certainly, many couples rejoice that the Pill exists. As another husband put it, "With my wife on the Pill, any moment is the right moment for love. No plans. No calculation. Unpremeditated sex is marvelous! We are in love, and it seems the right way for people in love to have sex."

But as the number of Pill users increased from hundreds of thousands to millions, evidence of another sort became evident. In a few instances, the Pill apparently was responsible for marital difficulties, not because of an effect on the wife, but because of a change in the husband's attitude.

I am often asked this question: why must the woman take a contraceptive pill and not a man? Indeed, it may seem strange that initial research was in the field of ovulation suppression rather than suppression of sperm development. It might be argued that accomplishing the former is so much easier than the latter, and, furthermore, that ovulation suppression had been utilized for years in the treatment of dysmenorrhea and endometriosis. However, those are not the reasons. It is generally accepted that the male is much more susceptible to psychological factors in his sexual activity than the female. With his virility and sense of maleness, his self-esteem is more closely allied to the sexual act than that of a woman. Impotence is far more debilitating psychologically to the male than frigidity is to the female. Although he usually plays the aggressor's role in sexual relations, he is extremely sensitive to even slight affronts to his masculinity. For all these reasons, it has been assumed that any method of contraception that diminished sperm count would create psychological problems for many men, which might lead to ego loss and impotence. Women, more pragmatic about sex, fail to ovulate and never miss it unless they fail to menstruate. Since bleeding may occur in the absence of ovulation, no major physical change is evident.

In the early days of clinical investigation with the Pill, the husband was almost completely ignored. The development of "husband factors" arose subsequent to closer study of the family unit and specific complaints from unhappy wives. This unforeseen aspect of the Pill emphasizes the great importance of psychological factors affecting sexual relationships between men and women.

The major problem develops when a previously normal wife

notes a marked increase in libido. This usually is the direct result of removal of fear of pregnancy. She enjoys intercourse more, wishes to engage in it more frequently, acquiesces more willingly, and occasionally may demonstrate aggressiveness about obtaining it. I should point out that, whereas this may seem idyllic to many husbands (at least temporarily), to others it engenders frustration, worry, fear, and occasionally impotence.

Apparently some husbands are pleased when their wife refuses to have intercourse. It must be a "game people play." The husband suggests sex, becomes aggressive, complains when his wife is unwilling, but is secretly pleased and possibly relieved when she is uninterested. A typical case, cited by Dr. M. J. Meldman, a Chicago psychiatrist, in a professional journal, *Psychosomatics,* is that of an ebullient salesman who enjoyed all the superficially manly activities: fishing, hunting, drinking, following sports avidly. He thought of himself as a sexually virile individual and blamed his frail, nervous wife because they had intercourse only about once in every six weeks. Finally, he urged her (despite their Catholicism) to start the Pill, not worry about pregnancy, and "to relax and enjoy it." She began the Pill, and she did stop worrying. More important, she began to enjoy sexual relations for the first time in her life. Unfortunately, this libidinous aspect of the Pill was not reflected in the behavior of the husband. Intercourse occurred, as before, once in six weeks.[42]

English physicians have reported that husbands of Pill users are complaining that their wives are "flat," meaning they no longer have the customary variation in desire. Many husbands have stated that they prefer their wives unpredictable, sometimes refusing, sometimes demanding. There are many men, apparently, to whom variety of response is appealing.

The problems are compounded for some men if the wife becomes more sexually aggressive. Dr. Meldman has speculated that the liberating effect of the Pill on the wife evokes all the latent emotional and sexual immaturity in the husband, once he is faced with real demands on his sexuality. Sexual aggressiveness by the female, while known in the animal kingdom, may produce a regressive attitude in the male *homo sapiens*. Wives have complained to me about their impotent husbands who developed this difficulty only after they started on the Pill. They complained that their husbands would become sexually aroused when they undressed before them, only to lose their erection if they assumed the dominant role in the sex act or became the least bit animalistic.

Dr. Joseph Garai, a psychologist, believes certain characteristics of married sex in the United States should be kept in mind when usefulness of the Pill is evaluated.[43] He stresses the American preoccupation with sexual performance. This, he believes, has had the effect of putting husbands and wives on trial before each other to prove their sexual worth. "Competition has spread from the business world to the bedroom, where it doesn't belong," he says; and he cautions further, "The destructive effects of such sexual competition on the marriage union can't be cancelled by the Pill. People need to be taught the best uses of contraceptives, just as they need to learn the best uses of sex, too."

One couple cited by Dr. Meldman had a competitive sexual situation, although they didn't realize it until the wife started the Pill.[42] Previously, her frigidity supplied a target for his aggression —or pseudo-aggression, as it turned out. His complaints were that he never "got enough sex." Actually, he didn't want any more and was probably afraid of sex. When his wife started on the Pill and her frigidity disappeared, his defenses were exposed as were his hidden fears. An ideal situation is thus created for infidelity by the unsatisfied wife.

Another illustration is taken from the life of a busy young business executive.[42] One day he noticed dizzy spells during a conference. Similar spells began to occur at the commuter station and in restaurants. During the attacks, he noted a migraine-like throbbing and stiffening of the muscles of the back of the neck, not unlike the symptoms of women with acute anxiety or hysteria. As Dr. Meldman probed deeper into the executive's background, he found that his attacks began the day after his wife started taking the Pill. Soon after, the husband became impotent.

How could a man become impotent because his wife is taking a contraceptive which is supposed to improve the quality of their sexual relations? An answer comes from psychiatrist Ralph Greenson, who states he is not surprised by the sexual apathy of husbands whose wives take the Pill. "American men are becoming more and more lethargic in their sex lives anyway," Dr. Greenson says.

Dr. John MacLeod of the Cornell Medical Center has studied the effect of stress on the sperm count and found that the count is lowered by fatigue, tension, and worry—all ingredients of a stressful situation. In this light, consider the mental gymnastics, the cerebral furor of the husband engaged in nervous anticipation of an important board meeting, a face-saving sale, or a last-minute financial arrangement to meet an income tax deadline. He is mentally and physically spent—in no mood to satisfy his newly libidinous, Pill-taking wife. Combining the problems of stress with excessive smoking, overindulgence in alcohol, and the use of certain drugs such as amphetamines, the American male is lucky if he can effect an erection, much less maintain one. Or, perhaps the effects of nudity everywhere, bare legs, bare bosoms, and free love superimposed on a "temporarily sterile" but overly aggressive wife result in a "take it or leave it" masculine attitude. No longer the virile attacker, he becomes the docile partner rendering mere service to his peer—or at least he feels that way.

Occasionally, the husband's reaction may take the form of extreme jealousy, even to the point of paranoia. A case in point[42] is that of an extremely masculine football coach whose wife began taking the Pill after the birth of their fourth child. She enjoyed her newly found sexual freedom almost to the point of nymphomania. A few months later she detected a change in her husband's behavior. He became suspicious, surly, and even hostile, but his sexual interest waned. He suspected that, because of his wife's interest in sexual activity, there was nothing to prevent her from seeking satisfaction outside the marriage. After accusing her of "making a fool of him," he finally reached an emotional climax and beat her.

Such a change does not surprise Dr. Mary Calderone, Executive Director of the Sex Information and Education Council of the United States. She comments, "Present day contraception with its far less sexually obtrusive methods may sometimes serve to bring the patient face to face with her own sexuality or that of her husband—a confrontation that often results in anxiety or panic on the part of the husband or wife."[42]

Dr. Martin Loeb, Director of the School of Social Work at the University of Wisconsin, points out that the "roles have changed fast because of the new era of awakened sexuality. Traditionally the male has been seen as the protector of the dependent female."[42] This is not quite the case these days. Dr. Loeb cites a junior business executive who told his wife he was going to buy a new sports car. She replied that if he did, she would throw away her contraceptive pills. This was tantamount to her quitting her job, getting pregnant, and adding a host of expenses. He drove his old car.

Dr. Loeb believes that the Pill has removed the biological basis of the double standard. It unshackles the human spirit and provides a sense of equality for women. Dr. William Masters states, "To date, a sexual role for the female in which she freely participates has not received total acceptance in Western culture, despite the currently nebulous state of the double standard. The incredible swing from yesterday's Victorian repression to today's orgasmic preoccupation has taken the human female but a few decades."[44]

Women have long claimed their abilities far exceed the customary roles of wife, mother, and homemaker. Changes that began with the right to vote have occurred rapidly, for good and ill. Today's woman smokes, drinks, gets drunk, curses, runs businesses, drives taxis and trucks; she becomes an able lawyer, doctor, philosopher, artist, and political leader. The Pill, in a manner superior to previous contraceptives, enhances her opportunities to prove an equality of sexuality to dubious males.

Dr. Greenson, whom I quoted previously, has commented, "Woman power is just like black power and it's going to have a similar impact. Faced by the growing public effectiveness and independence of women, men have traditionally reacted as if their masculinity were under attack."[43] In consequence, Dr. Greenson said, "American men are beginning to show a preference for demure, passive women. Perhaps the golden day of the shy, purring Southern belle is due for revival."

Surely, the feminine mystique has left the bedroom. The heightened receptiveness and aggressiveness of a woman on the Pill unfortunately poses a problem for some men who achieve ego satisfaction from their sexual prowess and who cannot adjust to a changed sexual role for their wives.

Indirectly, at least, the Pill contributes to other marital problems. Because the Pill eliminates even accidental pregnancies, career wives are able to postpone families indefinitely. One husband complained about his wife, "She doesn't want children at all . . . won't even talk about having them."[43] He observed an unattractive selfishness in her. Obviously, if a wife wishes to continue working and enjoy the money, freedom, and self-esteem that result, she now has the capability to do so and there isn't much her husband can do about it. That this can lead to altered marital roles and stress is obvious.

The statement must be made about husbands, as it was about wives, that the Pill is no panacea for marital and sexual incompatibility. The Pill is an excellent solution for the problem of contraception. It may secondarily increase a wife's sexual desire, but there are no ingredients in the Pill that alleviate male-female competition or marriage stress. Furthermore, as far as I know, there are no magic remedies that will permit a husband to satisfy his wife's desires beyond his usual capabilities. Were such a medication available, it would outsell the Pill a thousand times.

In my opinion, the Pill poses a problem for only a minority of husbands and even then it exposes only those problems that were latent in the marriage. But there is still a silver lining to the dark cloud hovering over those husbands who become impotent, suspicious, or violent when their wives use the Pill. By facing the problem directly and by making needed adjustments, happier marriages and improved sexual relations are possible. Psychotherapy may be necessary for severe maladjustments, but even in psychotic individuals, modern therapeutic concepts have proved corrective and complete cures are possible. For most couples, frank and open discussion of individual attitudes is necessary. If the husband is willing to accept his wife's changed role in sexual relationships and if she is able to appreciate her husband's sensitivity to psychological factors, a complete and happy reunion is usually possible. Husbands and wives who are forced to come to terms with their own sexuality may well end up with a more mature marital relationship.

In any event, the risk that the husband may regress sexually is not, in the opinion of most doctors, a valid reason to withhold the Pill.

21. Brave New World: The Future of Contraception

ANY DISCUSSION of the psychological, moral, and social effects of the Pill must consider the future of contraception. At present, the Pill, although a distinct improvement over earlier methods of contraception, is actually quite primitive when compared to contraceptive methods that might be developed.

It is not science fiction to suggest that within the next decade pregnancy may be prevented for periods of three, six, twelve and even twenty-four months with a single "shot"; that wives may be immunized against their husbands' sperm or husbands against their own; that pregnancy may be controlled by taking a pill once a month or when needed. Research is proceeding to develop all of these methods.

Some time ago I suggested that the ideal method of birth control would be a negative one. Instead of the majority of women being able to conceive during the reproductive period of life, the situation would be reversed, and the majority of women would not be able to conceive unless a specific substance was added to or removed from the body's reproductive mechanism.

My suggestion, quite understandably, has elicited a variety of reactions. Dr. Joseph W. Goldzieher agrees with the concept, saying, "Although the Pill is virtually 100 per cent effective when used correctly, there are always people who are not aware of it, who are illiterate or simply not motivated to take the Pill." He adds, "They will continue to reproduce at the will of Nature. It would be much more compatible with human intelligence for women to be infertile at all times and, from a philosophical view, every child would be a wanted child."

Dr. Harry Rudel of the Population Council in New York City disagrees, saying my suggestion should be dated for 1984. "It's just too George Orwellian for us. I think it would be putting a lot of power in the hands of a few to decide who is going to have a baby. It would take away much of man's freedom of choice."

I cite my suggestion and the responses to it to make the point that scientific research, spurred by the threat of world overpopulation, seems destined within the next few years to give mankind the ability to control conception completely and efficiently. Whether such contraceptive techniques will be used or should be used are problems that individuals and society will have to decide.

Certain it is that the Pill is only the beginning. A great deal of research is underway to develop improved methods of contraception. The Ford Foundation has granted $18.7 million to scientists to search for "simpler, safer, more effective" ways to control human reproduction than now exists. "Despite their remarkable record, neither the presently available oral contraceptives nor intrauterine devices are ideal for all users," says McGeorge Bundy, President of the Foundation. He refers to studies showing that about half the women who begin using intrauterine devices stop after two years. He also cites reports that in undernourished women, some contraceptive pills produce excessive nausea and vomiting. "Thus the need remains," says Bundy, "to speed development of promising, but unexploited methods from which basic research has been completed, to accelerate research on others, and to continue basic investigation in reproductive biology that may yield further practical approaches. Equally urgent is the need to continue evaluation and improvement of present methods."

All of the major investigators receiving grants from the Ford

Foundation are working with monkeys, whose cyclic reproductive pattern resembles that of humans. The largest grant, $1.6 million, was awarded to the Bio-Medical Division of the Population Council to establish a new monkey colony for contraceptive research at the Rockefeller University in New York City. Research there is being concentrated on development of "morning after" pills and implanted progestins that filter slowly into the body and prevent conception for long periods of time.

A grant of $846,000 went to the University of Pennsylvania, where Dr. Luigi Mastroianni, a pioneer investigator of intrauterine devices, will seek to improve our understanding of how the IUD works and how this method may be improved. The new grant will permit doubling of the monkey colony to about three hundred animals and support continued training of young people in research on reproductive biology.

The sum of $990,000 was awarded to Yale University School of Medicine. A Foundation spokesman noted that the Yale monkey colony is especially valuable because it has existed for years, enabling several generations of simians to be studied. Under the direction of Dr. John Morris, Professor of Obstetrics and Gynecology, Yale researchers will investigate new oral contraceptives, including several compounds that they believe may be effective "postcoital" pills.

Similar compounds will also be tested at the Cornell University Medical Center in New York City. It received a grant of $930,000 for a program directed by Dr. Fred Fuchs, Chairman of the Department of Obstetrics and Gynecology. In addition to "morning after" pills, Dr. Fuchs will investigate slow-release implants and the ability of various compounds to act on substances found in the Fallopian tubes and on intrauterine muscle activity to prevent fertility.

Besides these major grants, the Foundation is channeling support to basic and applied research in sixteen other institutions in the United States and abroad. Bundy expressed the hope that in the future the National Institutes of Health would devote a larger share of its funds to research on contraceptives. Private sources can only hope to drive an opening wedge in man's knowledge.

Full development can come only with extensive efforts supported by public funds.

A logical question is, "Why seek an improved contraceptive, if the Pill is 100 per cent effective?" No one claims that the Pill, either now or ever, is perfect. Compared to previous methods of contraception it may be marvelously sophisticated; compared with what is to come, it must be regarded as a useful, but crude advance. The Hellman Committee, in its report to the Food and Drug Administration in 1967, stated flatly, "Oral contraceptives currently in use are probably not those that will be employed ten or even five years hence."

The major flaw in the Pill is the fact that the very completeness of the protection it provides sometimes adds its own unique burden to the feminine nerves—by making forgetfulness inexcusable. There is no doubt that the Pill works, and physicians know well how it works, but it is effective only if taken each day for twenty or twenty-one consecutive days each month. If a user forgets one, two, or, at most, three days, the effect is lost for the month and pregnancy may occur.

"Of course, anyone can learn to count to 20, even illiterates," a woman physician has said, "but women of all social and educational levels have very human lapses." It is difficult sometimes to remember to take one colored pill for fifteen mornings, next a different-colored pill for five more, then none for a period of time, and finally to begin again on a specific day, which is the regimen imposed by the sequential pills. The most difficult task for most women is remembering whether she actually took the Pill the previous day. Some women cannot remember whether they took the wash to the laundry the day before, so it is not surprising for them to forget such an effortless action as swallowing a pill. Obviously, the consequences of not taking a pill are of greater magnitude than having forgotten a husband's shirts. The result, at least in certain tense individuals, is that the subconscious mind strains twenty-four hours a day to keep track of a simple schedule. I have known patients in whom insomnia was due to their inability to remember whether they had taken that day's pill as soon as the interlude of intercourse was over.

Other disadvantages are the side effects and the complications of the Pill. Smaller doses and new compounds have made the side effects minimal, compared to five years ago. Still, some users do experience abnormal bleeding, digestive upsets, excessive weight gain, skin problems, dizziness, mental depression, or decreased libido. The major complications, blood clotting and embolism, occur rarely and must be compared with the risks of not using the Pill. The incidence of thrombosis and embolism has not been determined in users of mini-dose regimens. Present evidence suggests that it will be insignificant. I doubt whether the cancer riddle will ever be solved, since the newer agents will replace the Pill before prolonged use becomes a reality. Even though only a small minority of women have these difficulties, search continues for a method of contraception that eliminates the side effects entirely.

Although research is aimed at developing *an* ideal contraceptive, it is more likely that several will be marketed. As McGeorge Bundy has said, "There is never likely to be one perfect pill for all individuals," but a variety of approaches. Research is progressing on several fronts, each of which has particular merit. Major efforts are directed toward: (1) refining the Pill to reduce side effects; (2) developing an everyday pill; (3) using injectable hormones; (4) perfecting a "morning after" pill; (5) improving intrauterine devices; (6) producing anti-fertility vaccines; and (7) making compounds safe to control sperm production in the male.

REFINEMENTS IN THE PILL

In the last half of 1967, several pills were made available with lower dosage in an effort to reduce side effects. The first of these was Ovulen, which contained only 1 mg. of a very potent progestin, ethynodiol diacetate, plus .1 mg. of the usual estrogen. Other manufacturers soon followed, the next preparations being Ortho-Novum-1, Norinyl-1, and Norlestrin-1. These contain only 1 mg. of progestin (compared to 2 mg. or 2.5 mg. in the prior preparations) and only .05 mg. of estrogen (half the former dosage). These agents are just as effective in conception control as the higher doses. However, because of the low amount of estrogen in these mini-dose pills, breakthrough bleeding is more common. Patients taking the mini-pill may have to double the dose frequently until the endometrium adapts to this estrogen level.

One possible solution to the problem of breakthrough bleeding is to increase the amount of estrogen up to .2 mg., and markedly reduce the progestin. In studies now underway, the progestin has been reduced to .5 mg. or even .1 mg. This avoids the marked anti-estrogenic effect that newer, more potent progestins have on the endometrium. Clinical studies are now underway in Egypt, Mexico, and other countries to test such preparations. An ideal progestin would not be anti-estrogenic, would aid in suppressing ovulation, produce regular withdrawal bleeding, and have no side effects. Such a progestin is not available.

THE EVERYDAY PILL

Several attempts are being made to simplify the regimen of oral contraceptives by having the patient take a pill continuously.

Already on the market is Noriday, developed by Syntex, which is packaged as twenty-eight pills. The first twenty-one pills are the mini-dose Norinyl-1, containing 1 mg. of progestin and .05 mg. of estrogen. The remaining seven pills are inert "duds" or "placebos." These are taken during the days when the patient menstruates. This system, it is hoped, will eliminate the problem of the user forgetting to resume taking her pills after menstruation. Presumably, other pharmaceutical houses will soon market similar systems.*

Another regimen presently being tested is the constant sequential method. This system, presently called Profem, simulates to a certain extent the gradually increasing level of estrogen during the proliferative phase of the cycle and the second surge of estro-

* Parke-Davis has just marketed Norlestrin 28-1 (each yellow tablet contains 1 mg. of the progestin [norethindrone acetate] and .05 mg. of an estrogen [ethinyl estradiol]; plus 7 white, inert tablets). Searle has just released Ovulen-28 of which the first twenty-one tablets are the usual combination, the next seven "dummies."

gen and progesterone after ovulation. Pills 1 through 7 contain only .025 mg. of estrogen, while the next fifteen pills contain .1 mg. of estrogen. Since only .07 to .08 mg. is necessary to suppress ovulation, the patient is protected against conception after the first week. During the last seven days of the constant cycle, a pill containing .125 mg. of estrogen is combined with 10 mgs. of a synthetic progestin known as Provera. The day following pill 28, pill 1 is taken. Because of the lowered dose of estrogen, a withdrawal flow usually occurs in two or three days. This system offers complete conception control, because it is most unlikely that ovulation will occur during the first six or seven days of the cycle. Furthermore, the woman is usually menstruating during this time. The regimen does away with "memory testing," and, in my opinion, seems an ideal preparation for the premenopausal patient. A further advantage is the elimination of seven days of each month of estrogen insufficiency during which time complaints are frequent.

A different approach to an everyday pill is now being clinically evaluated. If approved for public use, it will be a significant advance in oral contraception. The Pill contains no estrogen, thus eliminating all the untoward side effects of this hormone. According to the April, 1968, report of the *British Medical Journal*, estrogen, not progestin, was indicted as the culprit responsible for the increased incidence of thromboses and embolism. In the "mini-pro-solo" (small doses of progestin only) pill, we can finally dispose of this major disadvantage of the Pill. Moreover, "mini-pro-solo" does not usually interfere with ovulation, thereby eliminating one of the major disadvantages of the current pill. Finally, the system aids the memory problem.

Each pill contains only a tiny dose of synthetic progestin. Studies in Mexico City and other areas are using .25 to .5 mg. of the progestin chlormadinone (the progestin presently used in the last five days of C-Quens) or norethindrone (the progestin in Ortho-Novum, Norinyl, Norlestrin, and other brands).

The exact mechanism of action of this everyday progestin Pill is not known. Endocrine studies have shown that most women do ovulate. Only about 22 per cent of those tested have failed to ovulate, probably because of an individual sensitivity to the progestin. Since ovulation occurs, pregnancy is prevented by one or more of the following methods: (1) by changing the cervical mucus to make it unreceptive to sperm; (2) by altering the endometrium both in appearance and function so that a normally fertilized egg will not implant; (3) by speeding the delivery of the fertilized egg through the tube and into the uterus. In animals, estrogen slows the delivery process of eggs to the uterus; synthetic progestins may accelerate it. Since the fertilized egg usually spends about three days in the tube and another three days floating in the cavity of the uterus, it is possible that "early delivery" would result in an inhospitable reception so the egg is cast out in menstruation.

Since most women have a normal ovulation under this system, one would expect that a normal amount of estrogen and progesterone would be secreted following ovulation and that the endometrium would go through its usual development. That this does not occur is probably an effect of the anti-estrogenic effect of the progestin. This is also the probable cause of the breakthrough bleeding that occurs in 20 per cent of the patients. There is some change in cycle length, apparently caused by specific endocrine changes affecting ovulation. Four per cent of the patients who previously had regular menstrual cycles experienced cycles shortened to between twenty-one and twenty-four days. About 20 per cent of those tested had cycles of between thirty-six and fifty-nine days. Only 65 per cent had a normal cycle of twenty-five to thirty-five days. A report from the studies in Mexico City utilizing .5 mg. of chlormadinone without estrogen indicated a pregnancy rate of 3.7 per cent.

A recent report by Dr. Elizabeth Connell of New York[45] indicated that the "mini-pro-solo" pill *did not* block ovulation in 78 per cent of the patients studied; *did not* increase the risk of clotting and thromboses (this was borne out in animal studies, as well); and *did not* increase a specific enzyme, alkaline phosphatase, which is highly elevated in both pregnancy and "regular pill" users. There were 18 unplanned pregnancies in 859 patients, 12 resulting from method failure. Three planned pregnancies occurred within one to three months following cessation of medication.

Despite assumptions that the mini-dose program would be virtually self-regulating in the face of formidable educational and language barriers, Dr. Connell found a high incidence of unreliability to be characteristic of the clinic population. Only one-third of the first one hundred patients who claimed that they had taken the pill properly actually proved to have done so when their precounted pill supply was checked. One-third had taken too many, and one-third had taken too few.

Dr. Connell concluded, "We don't know how or why it [the experimental progestin pill] works in such a high percentage of patients. Low dosage progestagens may produce less suppression of the pituitary, but I think there is evidence that it also interferes with the biochemistry of the individuals taking it."

In this study, the effectiveness of the mini-pill was comparable to that of the IUD, but not as good as that of the conventional combined or sequential oral pills now in use.

Although the concept of estrogen-free, uniform, daily medication appeared to offer many advantages over the conventional pill, bleeding irregularities persisted in 23 per cent of the patients in Dr. Connell's study. Now investigators are around full circle to where they were ten years ago, advising addition of an estrogen to control the bleeding, but in an amount small enough to permit regular ovulation.

LONG-ACTING INJECTIONS

Extensive research in the development of injectable and long-acting agents for suppression of ovulation has been completed and is now before the FDA for study and approval. Such preparations have several advantages. The cumbersome process of Pill taking is eliminated. There is no problem of forgetfulness, and the psychological effects of Pill taking do not exist. Contraception is vastly easier, particularly in underdeveloped nations where illiteracy rates are high and the populace is accustomed to receiving medication by needle.

The injectable hormonal compound that has been clinically studied the longest is Deladroxate, a combination of long-acting progestational and estrogenic substances. The injection must be given within twenty-four hours before menstruation or on the eighth day following the onset of menstruation. Clinical investigation by various groups throughout the United States has indicated an efficacy of virtually 100 per cent. The side effects of the injection are about the same as with the Pill and the momentary discomfort of the needle is soon forgotten.

While it is extremely important for women to have the usual and regular breast and pelvic examinations by a physician, there is no need for monthly visits to the doctor to receive the injection of Deladroxate. Either the patient or her husband may administer the injection in the same way that insulin is administered to diabetics. However, because of the volume of the substance injected, the needle must be inserted into the muscular tissue of the buttocks. Preliminary instruction by a nurse or physician will prevent difficulties of administration.

The monthly injection of estrogen and progestin works exactly in the same way as the Pill, that is, by inhibiting ovulation. Some irregularity of cycles has been reported because of the long action of both hormones, and the usual incidence of breakthrough bleeding has been observed. Nonetheless, the system, if approved by the FDA, promises to be a major advance in contraception.

Even longer-acting injections are under study. The preparation used most commonly is Depo-Provera, a very potent and long-acting progestin which I have worked with since 1960. The effect of Depo-Provera on endometrial cancer, even when it has spread to the lungs and bone, has been described. I have also used Depo-Provera in treating patients with endometriosis, particularly those who could not tolerate the estrogen in most of the pills. In such patients I give 50 mg. of Depo-Provera every two weeks for four doses, then 200 mg. once a month for a year to create a pseudopregnancy. Since Depo-Provera has no estrogenic effect, the endometrium is not well maintained, and breakthrough bleeding is common during pseudopregnancy. Furthermore, the estrogen from the ovary is suppressed by the action of Depo-Provera. To offset the marked estrogen deprivation, small doses of estrogen may be given until the breakthrough bleeding stops. The effect of Depo-Provera is so prolonged that ovulation sometimes does not return for twelve to twenty-four months after cessation of this therapy. None of the patients treated by this method became pregnant during Depo-Provera administration, although a good number conceived shortly after recurrence of ovulation. In some patients it was necessary to use Clomid to expedite the return of ovulation.

Depo-Provera has a threefold effect and a number of other advantages. First, it is a "neuter" progestin, that is, it does not possess estrogenic or androgenic (malelike) side effects. Second, it is an excellent inhibitor of the pituitary, and therefore prevents ovulation. Depo-Provera's action is more potent than that of the Pill, reducing ovarian hormones to a minimum. (The effectiveness of the Pill depends initially upon the estrogen which reduces, but does not completely inhibit, FSH and the progestin that suppresses the mid-cycle peak of LH, whereas the basal excretion of LH does not seem to be affected. Prolonged administration of estrogen alone, as well as with added progestin, results in a markedly diminished secretion of both FSH and LH.)

Depo-Provera has other advantages. The cervical mucus is diminished because of the anti-estrogenic effect of the drug, thus preventing sperm migration into the uterus. The endometrium is prevented from attaining normal growth; thus, any egg that might become fertilized will not implant. Abnormalities of the endometrium, such as hyperplasia, are averted. Patients with severe breast pain as a result of estrogen-progestin stimulation note marked improvement after Depo-Provera because of its anti-estrogenic effect.

Depo-Provera is being tested as an anti-conception agent in numerous centers in the United States and by Dr. Juan Zanartu in Santiago, Chile. Doses vary between 150 mg. every three months, 500 mgs. every six months, to 1,000 mgs. yearly. Although it is much too early to accept this as a perfected method of conception control, the number of pregnancies reported has been extremely small. The major problem seems to be breakthrough bleeding, but this may be controlled by judicious use of an oral estrogen.

Dr. Edward Tyler of the University of California has recently reported his results of 216 women who were given 150 mgs. of Depo-Provera by injection every three months.[46] No pregnancies occurred in 2,150 women-months of use. The major problems with this regimen were irregular bleeding or total absence of a menstrual pattern. But Dr. Tyler was using a new concept in hormonal contraception. In other types that have been used systemically, including the once-a-month injection, there has been an attempt to maintain the normal menstrual pattern. In Dr. Tyler's series, some women bled at intervals of three days, whereas others would go as long as 146 days before bleeding again. Some women bled for a single day, others for fifty days or more.

Dr. Tyler stated that the patients in his program demonstrated a "good deal of motivation." Only 5.5 per cent discontinued the program because of bleeding problems. The women in this study had already turned down "once-a-month" injections because they preferred less frequent injections; they had turned down all kinds of pills, intrauterine devices, and vaginal methods. In a group of twenty-nine patients who discontinued the Depo-Provera injections, one-third resumed ovulation within six months, and all had ovulated by the end of one year.

It has become clear to investigators that other progestins besides those used in Deladroxate and Depo-Provera could be utilized by injections, if some method were available for their gradual diffusion into the body. Dr. Sheldon Segal of the Population Council in New York has tested a silicone rubber capsule filled with progestin and placed under the skin. The progestin used was chlormadinone, a potent anti-estrogenic preparation that is similar to Provera, but with increased potency.

The capsule, made of Silastic, is manufactured by Dow Corning and is the same substance we use in surgical reconstruction of the Fallopian tubes. The material is completely harmless to the body tissues and is therefore an integral component of most artificial heart valves. The porosity of the capsule can be varied to regulate the rate of diffusion of the progestin and the length of its effectiveness. If the user were to become pregnant or wished to become so, the physician could easily remove the capsule from the skin.

Testing has progressed favorably in animals, but research has just reached the point of human clinical trials. Dr. Segal says, "It will take another two to five years to determine how well this method works." On the other hand, Dr. Howard Tatum, Associate

Director of the Population Council, recently announced that the "Implant," as it is called, will be available within a year or two.[47] Tatum called the Implant a head-on, broadside attack on the world's population explosion. "The Implant," says Tatum, "will be safe and reliable with no side effects." It will doom the Pill; millions of women will throw away their IUD's. There will be no estrogen in the Implant, doing away with nausea, weight gain, and depression. The progestin in the Implant is minimal, so that ovarian function is normal and ovulation occurs regularly.

The Implant capsule is about an inch long and as narrow as a piece of spaghetti. It is inserted with a hypodermic needle high on a woman's inner thigh. There is no pain since a local anesthetic is used. The capsule does not become imbedded in tissue and is therefore easily removed. At the end of the year the capsule can be removed, either through a suction technique with a needle or by making an incision and then pulling it out. If the Implant proves to be successful, the time span can be lengthened from one year to three years or five years by using "piggyback" capsules. It is possible that one might even be constructed that would be effective for a woman's entire reproductive span.

The method sounds almost too good to be true, but if it lives up to the advance billing, millions of women will heave a sigh of relief. I can see several areas for difficulty, however. First, the progestin used is essentially that reported by Dr. Connell, and both breakthrough bleeding and diminished efficacy were noted in her study. The Implant solves the problem of Pill taking, but I wonder if its anti-estrogenic effect will permit regular cycles to occur. Secondly, some women seem to develop a sensitivity to progesterone and progestins. They might reject the Implant. Thirdly, certain side effects are undoubtedly due to the progestin and these might negate the continued use of the Implant.

Dr. Tatum feels that "It's a simple matter for an American woman to go to the corner drugstore for her supply of pills. But in the underdeveloped regions of Asia, Africa and South America, women are often miles away from birth control stations, and it may take them days or weeks to get there. Besides, they are too busy fighting hunger to time their pills correctly."

When the Implant is ready for worldwide distribution, medical caravans operated by local governments could visit the remote villages and settlements just once a year.

Dr. Harry Rudel of the Population Council is experimenting with a method of contraception that works on the same principle as Dr. Segal's, but utilizes a different technique. Instead of a capsule, Dr. Rudel is experimenting with "micropellets," extremely tiny doses of hormone mixed with an adhesive material that controls the release of the drug. The advantage of this method, Dr. Rudel says, "would be the ease of administration using a hypodermic needle instead of an implantation procedure." The disadvantage is that there is at present no way to reverse the process if the user wished to become pregnant or, worse, did become pregnant. The patient would just have to wait until the dose had been completely used. It is quite possible, however, that some agent might be developed that would negate the effect of the hormones in the pellets.

One of the difficulties with any of the long-acting progestins, whether given by the injection or in implanted capsules or injected micropellets, is that regular menstrual periods, as women know them, might not occur. If the progestin is kept at a very low level, ovulation and menstruation should occur normally. In some susceptible women, however, the progestin might be so potent that bleeding would not occur at all.

I have repeatedly emphasized to my patients and to audiences to whom I talk that menstruation serves no useful purpose. Menstruation is simply the result of *not* getting pregnant—nothing more. There is no evidence that menstruation cleanses the body of poisons or anything else. The fact that some women feel better after a menstrual flow cannot be denied, but this is an effect of the hormonal changes that have occurred in the ten days to two weeks prior to the menstrual flow, not of the bleeding. Avoidance of these peaks of hormonal activity will remove the symptoms associated with what is generally called "premenstrual tension."

In my experience I have found that women can accept the absence of menstrual periods—and be happy to be rid of the monthly "curse"—if the facts are explained to them. Doing this on a mass basis, however, would be an immense education problem, particularly among the less educated. In certain races, mystique and superstition are associated with menstruation. Not only does the notion that menstruation cleanses the body persist, but also the idea that monthly bleeding is a mark of femaleness and desirability. I've had patients whose lives depended upon hysterectomies beg me to "leave the uterus in," because their "man" would no longer consider them women if they didn't bleed. Such attitudes, however widespread they may be, are an obstacle to be overcome in any worldwide program of population control.

POSTCOITAL, OR "MORNING AFTER," PILLS

In 1966, Dr. John Morris and Dr. Gertrude Van Wagenen of the Yale University School of Medicine reported their studies with the "morning after" pill at the annual meeting of the American Fertility Society. Needless to say, their report created quite a stir among the members of the press and the lay audience. Even the suggestion that it might be possible for a woman to swallow a pill *after* intercourse, rather than taking them for twenty days, and prohibit pregnancy proved rather exciting.

The gynecologists and clinical investigators who heard the presentation of Drs. Morris and Van Wagenen were interested, but they did not react with the excitement exhibited by the press. The report described tests performed on several women, most of them rape victims. They were given the familiar synthetic estrogen DES (diethylstilbestrol) for five days after intercourse in doses of 50 to 100 mgs. This is fifty to one hundred times the usual dose, and the patients, quite predictably, exhibited severe nausea and vomiting. None of the patients became pregnant, *presumably* because the estrogen altered the endometrium to prevent the fertilized egg from implanting.

But the size of the dose and the nausea produced were not the principal reservations about this method. The unknown fact is whether any of the patients were indeed pregnant! Medical science has no way of discovering, at this time, whether an egg has been fertilized that soon after intercourse. Dr. Celso Garcia of the University of Pennsylvania, speaking before the Planned Parenthood Association of California in 1967, made this comment about the "morning after" pill: "One has to consider that very few cycles of observation and very few patients have been reported. We know that in the average couple, there is about a 20 to 25 per cent chance of pregnancy occurring in any given cycle. So the fact that pregnancies have not been demonstrated in these women is not remarkable, and therefore we must not take a premature view that this is an acceptable method of treatment at this time." Dr. Morris quite agreed and suggests that this method be used only in emergency situations.

Dr. Morris and Dr. Van Wagenen are continuing their research by using other chemical agents in animal experiments. One compound used in studies with monkeys is ORF-3858. Early results of these studies have been highly encouraging, yet there are theoretical problems that concern us if the drug is to be used in humans.

ORF-3858 is the end product of extensive research, both at Yale and at the Worcester Foundation of Experimental Biology, where the late Gregory Pincus pioneered in the investigation of progestins. Many similar compounds were screened, but none was adequate to produce the desired effect. Some compounds were effective in one laboratory animal but not in others. Allied substances were ineffective in preventing pregnancy, but produced deformed offspring. Obviously, this is a major consideration in any postcoital preparation. Not only must it be 100 per cent effective in preventing pregnancy, but if it is not and should pregnancy occur, it must have absolutely no effect upon the fetus. At this writing, ORF-3858 is the first compound to prove safe and effective in every way in the monkey experiments.

No one is certain how ORF-3858 acts to force expulsion of the fertilized egg. One theory is that it produces contractions of the uterus that prevent the egg from implanting. Another possibility is that the compound acts on the Fallopian tubes, speeding the egg along so that it reaches the uterus prematurely. If the latter theory is correct, the drug's mechanism would be similar to that of a minidose progestin.

From Sweden comes a report of an even more startling drug

than ORF-3858. Unfortunately, the reports have appeared only in the popular press and not in the medical literature. The information presently available suggests that a drug, similar to clomiphene citrate, possesses a strongly anti-progesterone potential and has successfully induced a menstrual flow—and therefore an abortion —in pregnant women. According to reports, abortions have been successfully accomplished in women as late as the fourth month of pregnancy. If the information so far available is accurate, the drug acts by negating the vital functions of progesterone during pregnancy. The fertilized egg is held in the endometrium by progesterone. This hormone is vital for the supply of life-sustaining nutriments for the fetus. Any substance that negated progesterone could theoretically cause release of the contents of the uterus and abortion. There is, of course, the question of whether this compound produces abnormalities in the fetus if abortion does not occur. I will reserve comment on this preparation until an adequate number of patients have been reported in the medical literature.

Extensive research in the development of a postcoital pill is now underway. The reason is obvious: it may be used to protect a woman who has forgotten to take her conventional pill. This is a worldwide problem with the Pill, as exemplified by a report by Dr. John C. Cobb, Professor of Preventive Medicine at the University of Colorado. In describing the use of contraceptives in Pakistan, he said most of the oral contraceptives are being rejected. "Only eight or 10 of 2,000 women in the village have any schooling beyond the primary level," he reported. "Very few [women] ever believe that contraception might be possible. Lack of inclination to plan ahead, combined with ignorance make family planning unrealistic. Only those who plan ahead can use contraceptives effectively; so in each new generation the planners get fewer and the non-planners more numerous."

In those countries which have significantly reduced birth rates, abortion has been rather easily obtained. A do-it-yourself method of birth control, which could be used after pregnancy is suspected, would be more effective than contraception for those women who do not plan properly. If such a method proved to be 100 per cent effective, safe, cheap, and readily available to women throughout the world, its acceptance would be guaranteed.

If a pill were available that could be taken safely and effectively before the first missed menstrual period, it would have definite advantages over other methods. Since the woman would not know whether or not an egg had been fertilized, the pill could be taken with less guilt than would be involved with an abortifacient pill.

Dr. Gordon Perkins, Assistant Medical Director of Planned Parenthood-World Population, has cited the important advantages of the "morning after" pill. But he adds, "I wouldn't want this to be taken the wrong way—we are not for abortion. But this pill has the same advantage that abortion would have. If a woman finds she is pregnant, suddenly her motivation not to go through with that pregnancy can become very high, even though she may not have been motivated initially to use some precaution."

Development of a "morning after" pill has been slowed by a series of technical difficulties. In the first place, the designation as a "morning after" pill smacks of science fiction. It seems unlikely that researchers will devote much time developing a pill that a woman can pop in her mouth the morning after intercourse. Present plans for ORF-3858, the most promising of the postcoital drugs, call for administration of six pills, one a day, during the third week of the menstrual cycle. Once dosages are perfected, doctors believe they can reduce the pills to one to be taken near the end of the cycle. But this is hardly a "morning after" pill. It would be more accurate to speak of a "once a month" pill, the development of which may not be too many years away. My own guess is that the Implant of progestin will be available before the "morning after" pill, and the latter would be of importance only to the "occasional offender."

INTRAUTERINE DEVICES

Although the intrauterine device has been marketed for several years and used in millions of women, investigators still are seeking the method of action and are constantly modifying the unit to make it more effective. Present evidence suggests that the plastic coils and loops prevent conception by speeding the fertilized egg through the Fallopian tube in hours, instead of days, so that it arrives ahead of schedule and cannot implant on an "unripe" endometrium. Release of an endometrial "poison" is also a possibility.

The principal problem with the IUD as an effective contraceptive is that it does not remain in place. It may be extruded at the time of a menstrual period, silently and painlessly. On the other hand, pregnancies have occurred with the device in place, and several reports have described the device neatly tucked away in the membranes surrounding the baby at delivery. Another difficulty with the older devices is that one woman in five must have it removed because of discomfort or irregular bleeding. In some patients, the device has perforated the uterus and been found in the intestines.

Experimentation is underway to improve the method. One innovation developed in Denmark and now being tried in Pakistan is to construct the IUD in polygonal shape. This shape may adapt better to the intrauterine contour. Another experiment makes use of newer plastics. These are heated in warm tap water, then inserted into the uterine cavity. As the plastic attains the temperature of the uterus, it assumes the shape of the uterine cavity. Such a device may fill the nooks and crannies in the larger and irregularly shaped wombs, therefore affording greater protection against "fall out" and perforation.

Another system is to place the IUD in the uterus immediately following delivery or after a curettage for a miscarriage. Evidence suggests that the retention rate approximates 95 per cent by this method. Still another variation provides "double coverage." In this IUD, long-acting progestins are inserted and are gradually released. The latest method tested is a plastic ring containing Depo-Provera which is placed in the vagina (not the uterus) and, by gradually releasing the progestin, provides conception control.

REVERSIBLE SURGICAL STERILIZATION

In the past, numerous men and women have accepted surgical sterilization as a method of conception control. However, it has never been totally acceptable, particularly in the male, because of the possibility of permanent effect. In the female, the standard technique of dividing or tying off the Fallopian tubes is not always correctable. The same problem exists in the male when the vas deferens is tied. Although the surgical procedure in the male is a minor one and may be performed in the office of a urologist, ligation of the Fallopian tubes is a major abdominal procedure, except when it is done at the time of a Caesarian section.

In an effort to increase the reversibility of the operations, Dr. Hans Zinsser of the Columbia Presbyterian Medical Center in New York has injected liquid silicone rubber into the vas deferens of a few volunteer men. The substance solidifies in the tiny tubule of the vas and forms a plug that prevents passage of sperm. When fertility is desired, a simple surgical incision is made and the plug is removed. This method of reversible sterilization should be considered as an investigative procedure, since the long-term effects of silicone rubber on the lining cells of the vas deferens are unknown. Moreover, it is important to study the effects of this material on the formation of spermatozoa in the testicles before adopting it as an acceptable method of conception control.

Similar experiments have been performed utilizing the same silicone rubber in the Fallopian tubes. They have not been as successful, simply because the tube is larger and more tapered with a larger end near the ovary. Because of the natural contractions of the tube, the plastic plugs have been expelled. My own opinion of these methods is that they leave much to be desired in both a technical and physiological way, yet similar methods will be available for those who wish it. Dr. Shirodkar of India has devised a technique of folding and sewing the open end of the Fallopian tubes into a little pocket of tissue that lines the body cavity. If the woman subsequently desires pregnancy, the tube may be easily removed from its hiding place.

MALE CONTRACEPTIVES

Progress in developing "shots" and pills to control male fertility has lagged behind developments for the female. This is due, in part, to the fact that most authorities believe that conception control is a function of the female. Or, it may be due to the widespread belief that the presence of an adequate supply of sperm is of greater psychological importance to a man than ovulation is to a woman. Finally, the slow pace of research in the male may be due to the fact that investigators have found it difficult to separate sperm production from the process of male hormone formation.

Many previously tested chemicals have the property of diminishing or halting normal production of sperm. Some compounds even destroy the potency of sperm. An example is Enovid. Dr. Carl Heller administered this female contraceptive to male prisoners in Oregon. A marked change in the development of sperm cells occurred, but so did certain unwanted phenomena. The estrogenic potency of Enovid began to feminize some of the men, causing growth of breast tissue and reducing sex drive. Dr. Heller found that previously normal men began to tear down their calendars and other wall decorations featuring female nudity. This was sufficient warning to discontinue the administration of Enovid to males.

Several years ago another compound was tested. No feminizing effect occurred in volunteers, yet sperm counts were lowered. It seemed ideal, until doctors tried it on themselves. They were shocked to discover that drinking even small amounts of alcohol made their eyes turn fiery red, their faces flush, and their hearts pound. Some had excessive nausea and vomiting. Needless to say, a substance that is not compatible with alcohol in our present society is just not acceptable.

The same progestin mentioned previously, Depo-Provera, will suppress the sperm count in males, just as it suppresses ovulation in females. Apparently, Depo-Provera is effective because it suppresses the pituitary hormones necessary for normal sperm development. Dr. John MacLeod, Professor of Anatomy at the Cornell Medical Center, tested Depo-Provera in a prison farm in Arkansas. Although there is no doubt about the ability of this compound to suppress sperm development and diminish their motility, the question of reversibility without permanent damage still remains to be answered.

Recently an orally active drug that makes male animals temporarily infertile has been tested by Dr. R. J. Ericsson of the

Upjohn Company's biochemical research unit. This compound, 3-chloro-1, 2-propanediol, has been tested on rats, guinea pigs, and monkeys and is effective, as well as reversible, in all three. Apparently the drug affects sperm by rendering them incapable of fertilizing eggs, but it is neither spermicidal nor anti-spermatogenic. Furthermore, and most important, it does not affect libido. Dr. Ericsson has suggested that the mode of action may be to deprive sperm of their oxygen supply or allow the accumulation of metabolic wastes that make the sperm ineffective.

The psychological and physiological factors involved in the development of a chemical or hormonal agent for male contraception are so complex that researchers in this field are not optimistic about an early breakthrough. Eventually we may be able to inactivate sperm motility without affecting the hormonal milieu, the masculinity of the male. At the moment, such a method has not as yet reached the stage of clinical investigation.

ANTI-FERTILITY VACCINE

Most gynecologists feel that the science of immunology will be an increasingly important aspect in the treatment of female disorders in the future. Advances in this field have already permitted heart, liver, and kidney transplants. In the future, it may be possible for gynecologists to transplant ovaries, tubes, and even the uterus. Vaccines have been developed that build defenses against smallpox, poliomyelitis, and measles. Therefore, I look to immunization as the most attractive long-range hope for the creation of nonfertile states.

Theoretically, medical science should be able to produce immunity to fertility by sensitizing a man to his own sperm cells so that he produces antibodies that would inactivate them. Perhaps the same procedure could be carried out in the female so that she could be sensitized against her own egg cells. The obvious, and hopefully the simplest, method would be to desensitize a woman against her husband's sperm cells. It might even be possible to immunize the female against the male for a certain period of time, then the male against the female.

There is evidence at present to suggest that some women are infertile because of antibodies they have developed against their husbands' sperm. The only treatment for this unfortunate condition is continence (or use of a condom) for six months or more to prevent the sperm from coming in contact with the mucus of the cervix.

Dr. S. J. Behrman of the University of Michigan Medical Center has been conducting animal tests and experiments with human volunteers in an effort to produce antibodies. These antibodies, produced in the female, would cause sperm cells to clump together, lose their motility, and thus their ability to penetrate and fertilize an egg cell. Even if fertilization occurred, the presence of antibodies in the endometrium might prevent implantation of the fertilized egg.

Dr. Behrman has been successful in experiments in which the female rabbit was injected with a preparation made from a combination of reproductive tissues of male rabbits. These antibodies, produced in the females, completely prevented pregnancy. After the female had been sensitized, frequent intercourse restimulated the production of antibodies, keeping the level of immunity high. When Dr. Behrman used only seminal fluid (in which sperm cells are carried) and no spermatozoa, the results were equally good.

At the present time, Dr. Behrman and his associates are sorting out and identifying the chemical substances in the fluid which cause the antibodies to form. Thus, it is hoped that a very specific immunizing material may be found that may be of practical use. In studies of this type, it would be preferable to have a "short-term" rather than a "long-term" effect. This brings up the problem of "passive" versus "active" immunization. This is similar to the recent advances in the protection of RH-negative women against the red blood cells in their RH-positive fetus.

The ideal method of immunization would be to prepare antibodies against sperm in sensitized donor females and then inject only those antibodies into women not desirous of becoming pregnant. This is known as "passive" immunization, while "active" immunization would be similar to the familiar smallpox immunization. An important advantage is that the effect of the passive vaccine would wear away in a predictable length of time, whereas active immunization might last indefinitely.

Dr. Behrman has predicted that "We may have a very effective anti-fertility vaccine within five to ten years—possibly sooner with a little luck." This method would be the ultimate in conception control and probably the simplest. Recent progress in immunology suggests that rapid strides in the field are possible. Consider the heart transplants pioneered by Dr. Christian Barnard in South Africa and now performed in many hospitals. While much has yet to be learned, the fact the operations can be attempted indicates the progress in the field of immunology.

Just as the body has the ability to reject a transplanted heart, it might also have the ability to make a wife allergic to her husband so that every intercourse might bring a violent allergic reaction. Needless to say, this would defeat the basic purpose of the immunization, although it would no doubt result in fertility control.

Dr. Alan Guttmacher, President of Planned Parenthood-World Population, has commented, "Even though the progress made in the past decade has been magnificent, the prospects for the next five years are even more exciting." The need is urgent. Investigators are at work. Progress in the field of contraception is inevitable.

It is also inevitable that as new forms of fertility control are developed, new problems will emerge, compounding the social, moral, and psychological problems that already exist with the Pill. The present and future problems are the subject of subsequent chapters.

22. The Pill and the Teenage Girl

Since the Pill was developed over a decade ago, the idea has persisted that it encourages sexual promiscuity, particularly among teenagers. After all, the Pill is totally effective. If a teenage girl obtains a supply of pills and takes them correctly, she can use her body for pleasure without fear of pregnancy. A major bar to inchastity has been lowered. This, I believe, is a fear in the minds of many people. Is it justified?

This is a difficult matter for a physician to discuss, for it displaces him from medicine into morality. Moreover, the very nature of the subject is unscientific. Scientists demand "controlled" observations before concluding cause and effect. No scientist would design an experiment in which two or more variables existed if he were trying to determine the effect of only one. Thus, to conclude that the Pill is responsible for increasing sexual promiscuity in a world of nudity, pornography, alcohol, marijuana, and LSD borders on the ludicrous. Since the relationship of contraceptives to sexual morality cannot be evaluated with precision, it becomes obvious that many and varied opinions will demand attention. However, the opinion of a physician may be just as valid as that of a moralist or theologian.

Therefore, I will state my opinion before presenting those of others. I do not believe that fear of pregnancy has been a major deterrent to intercourse. Condoms and diaphragms have been readily available to those who desired "safe" intercourse. Furthermore, I do not believe that chastity before marriage is rooted in fear of pregnancy or disease, but in the moral fibers of the individual. In my opinion, the young people now participating in the "teenage copulation explosion" would have done so even if the Pill had not been developed. Looking toward the future, however, I do believe that the postcoital pill, when developed, may be an inducement to premarital sex.

There is another aspect of the problem which prevents collection of adequate and meaningful data. Whereas the total number of Pill users in the United States is known to be between 6 and 7 million, statistics are not available that divulge ages of the users. Furthermore, it is known that a certain amount of peddling goes on between over-twenty-one buyers and under-nineteen users. And other contraceptives have been available to teenagers for years, although it was usually a male function to provide the condom. But time and the Pill have brought about significant changes —that promote the acceptability of premarital sex.

Any discussion of premarital sex must begin with the word *promiscuous*. Properly defined, the word connotes lack of discrimination. A promiscuous girl copulates freely with almost anyone. There are such unfortunate individuals, but by any standards they are psychiatrically ill. They frequently become the heroine in today's best sellers or movies. A more correct term to apply to the problem under discussion is *premarital sex*, occurring between two young people who intend to marry or who have "gone together" long enough to develop emotional attachments. Indiscriminate, impulsive copulation without emotional involvement undoubtedly does occur, but in my opinion it is not as frequent as portrayed by the press. Behavior of this type may be ignited by drugs or alcohol, but I do not think it is induced by the Pill.

There is no doubt that a significant number of girls are engaging in premarital intercourse. A recent study among nearly all unmarried undergraduate women at Oberlin College, a select institution in a small town in Ohio with extremely high entrance

standards, showed that 40 per cent had engaged in sexual intercourse. One in thirteen had become pregnant, and 80 per cent of
the pregnancies were terminated by abortion.

What is the result of this change in mores? Which comes first,
the contraceptive or the changing code? Contraception in the
lives of teenagers has shifted from the shadows into the limelight
of their preoccupations. Dr. Mary Calderone has commented on
this correlation, "What has contraception to do with the teenager?
The answer is plain: the teenager is having sex, the teenage girl
is getting pregnant." I suppose one could add an observation that
those not taking the Pill are getting pregnant.

There is one question that is answered uniformly in the affirma-
tive in studies pertaining to sex, the Pill, and teenagers. "If you
knew that your teenage daughter was having regular intercourse,
would you prefer that she be given a supply of contraceptive
pills?" A few vindictive mothers state that pregnancy would "teach
her a lesson." None indicates that she approves of the arrangement; she merely accepts the lesser of two evils—the Pill and no
pregnancy is better than pregnancy and no pills.

The mores and morals in the vast majority of teenage girls have
fairly well jelled by the time the first opportunity for sexual intercourse appears. Fifteen or sixteen years of family experience and
parental guidance are usually adequate to establish firm moral
standards in most teenage girls. There is no doubt that this may
be buttressed by courses in sociology, family life, and sexual physiology and anatomy. It is obvious, however, that efforts to prevent
or curtail juvenile sex practices have been inadequate.

Urgency is the key word in education of contemporary youth
for sex, marriage, and parenthood. Consider the high incidence
of venereal diseases and illegitimacy among teenagers; of infant
mortality and illness; of criminal behavior; of destructive premarital sexual relations; of criminal abortion ending in death or
permanent infertility; of family instability, marital unhappiness,
and divorce.

Two of every five girls marrying are teenagers with an average
age of eighteen. In one study, half the high school girls getting
married were pregnant before the ceremony. The same study in-

creased the percentage to 80 when the husbands-to-be were high school boys. If these 80 per cent decided upon marriage *only* because of their state of pregnancy, would oral contraception have offered a preferable solution?

If these forced marriages were happy and permanent they might not be looked upon with disfavor. But figures provided by the U.S. Census Bureau indicate a divorce rate in teenage marriages three times higher than for those couples married between ages twenty-one and twenty-five. Other studies show that three of four teenage marriages end in divorce. Furthermore, within five years most of the partners in teenage marriages were engaged in adulterous behavior. Children born of teenage marriages are an unhealthy lot. A large percentage are underweight, premature, and sickly. Untreated syphilis in the mother, if it does not cause a miscarriage, damages the child for life. The death rate for infants born to teenage mothers has been estimated as high as 26 per cent.

The "teenage copulation explosion" has recently been investigated by a committee appointed by the British Medical Association. It concluded that there is an increased incidence of sexual intercourse among juveniles, together with a drop in the age of first experience, now usually between twelve and sixteen. They studied the sharp rise in illegitimate pregnancies, illegal abortions, and venereal diseases. For example, in England, "Sexually transmitted diseases have increased in recent years out of all proportion to population increase and, even more alarming, this increase is greater in the younger age groups." Between 1951 and 1962, the population increased by 6 per cent. But sexually transmitted disease increased 73 per cent. According to the World Health Organization, an increase in the incidence of syphilis ranged from 19 per cent in Canada to 85 per cent in Denmark. In the United States, the increase was 45 per cent.

Venereal disease is no longer restricted to prostitutes, Skid Row bums, or slum dwellers. It is rampant in scrubbed teenagers from middle- and high-income families. The age group from ten to twenty-four shows the highest incidence. Venereal disease affects adolescents and young adults on the average of one new case every two minutes . . . one of every thirty-five Americans under age twenty-five suffers . . . gonorrhea alone is fifty times more prevalent than polio . . . "In fact," says Dr. Frank J. Ayd, *"venereal disease is the most widespread adult communicable disease in the United States."*

There are numerous reasons given, other than oral contraceptives, for the VD explosion in teenagers. In metropolitan areas of prosperous countries, teenagers have less parental and adult supervision. They have more freedom, more money, plus easy access to salacious literature and movies. In addition, even adult attitudes toward sex, morality, and religion are changing; so are their opinions of premarital and extramarital sexual relations.

The British Medical Association Committee stated that the extent of promiscuous behavior can, to some extent, be assessed by the figure for illegitimate births, particularly among those in their teens. For example, two out of three babies born to girls under twenty years of age were conceived out of wedlock, and the total number of such births has doubled between 1948 and 1961. In the United States, the National Council on Illegitimacy recently reported that over 250,000 women bear children out of wedlock each year and about 90,000 of these are teenagers.

What will be the impact of the Pill in this teenage society? It has no protective effect against venereal disease, as does the condom. However, the protection it offers against illegitimate births, abortions, and ill-advised but forced marriages is of much greater magnitude. And modern sociologists, moved by compassion for the plight of unmarried teenage mothers, illegal abortions among them, the risk of high infant mortality, and severe obstetrical complications, are demanding that teenagers be protected from these hazards. It has been suggested that they be offered conception control both by advice and device. Most sociologists believe strongly that this service is "morally correct" and have urged that government pass laws which will establish family planning for teenagers.

Some countries are making changes in response to these suggestions. A new Danish "pregnancy hygiene" law went into effect in 1966. It authorizes any fifteen-to-eighteen-year-old girl to visit her own physician or a public clinic to be fitted with a diaphragm or get instructions in other contraceptive methods. Few objections have been raised publicly by parents or guardians.

The Dutch government is considering legislation that would liberalize laws regarding sales of contraceptives. This would reduce the minimum age from eighteen to sixteen. Great Britain is weighing a change in government policy recommended by the Family Planning Association that would permit unmarried applicants to receive advice on birth control.

The United States, through its Office of Economic Opportunity, has recently removed a former provision that forbade the use of grants to provide funds for contraceptive devices or drugs to unmarried women. Thus, local agencies have freedom to establish criteria for eligibility which are consistent with realistic local factors. The OEO policy attempts to provide communities with maximum flexibility in instituting measures to combat poverty according to self-determined needs and priority.

Meanwhile, some planned-parenthood clinics, local health departments, clinics with federal financial assistance, private physicians, and college student health services are providing birth control advice and/or materials for single American girls.

The medical profession has professed both pro and con opinions about providing contraceptives to unmarried girls. Dr. Frank J. Ayd recently polled prominent obstetricians, gynecologists, psychiatrists, and sex educators in an effort to ascertain their views on this subject. Their responses have been published in *Medical Science* in September, 1967. Some of the answers were:

Mary S. Calderone, M.D., Executive Director, Sex Information and Education Council of the U.S. (SIECUS):

> Those who want to instruct all 15-year-old girls in contraception are interested in preventing illegitimacy at any cost. There are others, however, who are convinced that the motivations for offering contraceptive services to an unmarried person under 18 must be made crystal clear, first to ourselves, then to her and last but not least to the public—including all other adolescents. I am convinced that this motivation must be a medical and health-based one; it must not depend on a desire to save welfare dollars, nor on a desire to control reproduction rates in specific social groups, nor even

merely on a desire to safeguard her against pregnancy. It must be an integral part of a medical judgment holistically arrived at as a part of a total therapeutic program that considers every aspect of her health needs: physical, mental and social. Then, if our judgment is that this individual's life pattern requires contraception, we cannot stop there, but must make sure that she is also helped towards the indicated therapy and rehabilitation, otherwise the contraception we give her, while certainly protecting her against pregnancy, will merely encourage her to continue, and even to expand, the socially-ill pattern of living that we know can, for her, end only in the destruction of herself as a unique and precious individual.

Elsie R. Carrington, M.D., Department of Obstetrics and Gynecology, Women's Medical College of Pennsylvania:

Those of us whose responsibilities include the care of young, unmarried mothers must certainly feel compassion for the distressing problems that the unwed mother, her family and the unwanted child must face. Surely, total medical care of these youngsters must include evaluation of their problems, counseling and, when necessary, institution of psychotherapy. In the meantime, it should be realized that a health hazard exists and that a safe method for protection against pregnancy is the proper and only humane treatment. So many of the teenagers we see in the prenatal clinic are neglected, unsupervised and uninformed. They constitute a high risk group, just as surely as the married mother with a serious medical disease. It seems reasonable to suggest that accurate information concerning contraception should not be given on a selective basis but should be an integral part of the sex education program for all adolescents in the high school curriculum. *I believe that the fear that this step would lead to promiscuity is wholly unfounded.*

Andre E. Hellegers, M.D., Department of Obstetrics and Gynecology, Georgetown University School of Medicine:

The offering of birth control information to unmarried, adolescent girls could be a matter of an individual physician's decision in a given case or one of general medical policy. In the former case, it would be impossible to say that one would never run into circumstances in which sure advice should be given. Viewed from the second point of view, i.e., as a general medical policy, several aspects should be considered. These have to do with technical and ethical aspects. The most frequent advocacy of such contraceptive advice is voiced in terms of preventing illegitimacy. Where previous pregnancy has occurred in an individual, and the intrauterine device (IUD) is therefore applicable in her case, effectiveness in preventing further illegitimacy can at least be reasonably expected. Where no previous pregnancy has occurred and the IUD is really not in the contraceptive arsenal, an entirely different situation exists. Many studies have shown that the use effectiveness of classical contraception (including daily pill taking) varies with motivation in the individual. It is unrealistic to expect that where intercourse occurs casually, the classical contraceptive methods are as effective as when they are used in a regular, predictable marital situation. Under such circumstances, the advocacy of contraception for the adolescent, never-married, never-pregnant girl, in my opinion, is likely to worsen the problem of illegitimacy. At a theoretical level, a sense of security exists which in practice is not achieved. At the level of the individual doctor-patient relationship, circumstances may arise, of course, in which this general rule would not pertain. It is obviously impossible *a priori* to exclude all women from such advice.

Dana L. Farnsworth, M.D., Director, Harvard University Health Services:

> I believe that birth control information should be made available to anyone who desires it, but that prescribing medication or equipment and supervising contraceptive practices of unmarried adolescent girls should not be done except after careful consideration of each girl's total situation, conference with parents or guardians, and consultation when appropriate with other vitally interested persons. There will be some situations in which supervision of contraception will be the least undesirable of all possible courses. In general, young persons will be helped most if their total needs are kept in mind and "disciplined and devoted delay" in beginning sexual relations is encouraged.

What is occurring among girls in their late teens and early twenties? What is the policy in our colleges? Nearly half of the nation's college health services now prescribe contraceptive pills, but only one in twenty-five will do so for single women who do not intend to marry in the near future. These findings, from 315 member institutions of the American College Health Association show: (1) 174 (55 per cent) do not prescribe contraceptive pills; (2) 77 (24 per cent) prescribe only to married women; (3) 23 (7 per cent) prescribe only for medical purposes; (4) 28 (9 per cent) will prescribe only for single women who take a premarital exam or show other intent to marry in the future; (5) 13 (4 per cent) will prescribe for single, unmarried women.

From Stanford University School of Medicine, Child Psychiatric Clinic, comes this statement by Dr. Beatrix Hamburg, Research Associate Psychiatrist:

> In part, the activist students who are loudly banging on the doors and asking to have a policy on "the Pill" are really asking to have an opinion expressed about the new morality. Whether we like it or not, a policy adopted by the student health service will be an implied administrative position. The issuance of pills or other devices on an open basis to any and all comers, without question, in a straight doctor-patient relationship will inevitably be interpreted by the students as a mandate for sexual freedom.
>
> It's important that any implied policy take into account a wide range of student needs. There are immature students who need the shelter and protection of a policy which protects them against a bandwagon effect, where undue pressure is put on these students to engage in sexual activities that they are not yet emotionally prepared for.
>
> At the same time, we have students who are at a stage where it is appropriate and they need elbow room to experiment. And we have other students who are extremely mature and are engaged in a monogamous, though not legally sanctioned relationship. All of these student needs are equally valid and need equal protection. It's important that student health services walk the tightrope in trying to meet all these varying needs.

What conclusions may be drawn from these opinions? The increasing demand for contraceptives by teenagers has posed a dilemma for the physician. Should he be a moralist and counsel chastity, or should he prescribe a contraceptive and leave morality to parents and religious leaders?

Dr. Frank Ayd has said that the views expressed in his survey of the leaders of the profession indicate that they generally hold a conservative position and do not favor providing contraceptives for unmarried teenagers. Physicians do not believe that making contraceptives available to young girls would solve the problem of illegitimacy. They agree with the view expressed by D. V. Van Emde Boas at the 1964 conference of the International Planned Parenthood Federation. "It is not contraceptives that they need," he said, "but a complete emotional re-education, to protect them from cheap and unsatisfactory adventures and against the self-punishment of pregnancy."

Stating my own view on the question of making the Pill available to unmarried teenagers, it must be obvious by now that I consider it a complex issue. I am not worried about physiological effects, since all of the individuals under discussion have established ovulation and adequate estrogen release. The estrogen effect on bone growth has already occurred. Nor am I particularly worried about producing a permanent derangement in the pituitary-ovarian axis that might lead to permanent sterility. For almost twenty years I have treated teenage girls with estrogenic substances to control acne, alleviate painful periods, and correct irregular bleeding. When the progestins became available in 1956, I began using the same compounds for these disease processes. These girls reestablished hormonal ovulation and menstruation as soon as the estrogen-progestin was discontinued. I cannot conceive of a logical reason, therefore, to expect deleterious long-range effects just because the Pill is now being used as an oral contraceptive—unless the latter is looked upon as something evil, something for which retribution is necessary.

Preventing illegitimacy is certainly to be desired, but compounding the problem of venereal disease is certainly *not* desired. Exploring the psychological factors affecting the girl, her partner, and the unwanted child that may result leads to the conclusion that all may be helped or harmed by the Pill. The social factors, considering the importance of a stable family unit in our society, would certainly favor prescription of the Pill. Legal factors, including the danger of malpractice suits against the physician prescribing the Pill, argue against its prescription.

The prevailing point to me, as I sift through all the pros and cons, is that the Pill will not solve all problems for all people. If we were dealing with a mentally retarded girl or someone who grew up on a desert island unexposed to civilization, the Pill would seem the only humane thing to do. But we are not dealing with such people. Today's copulating teenager may be foolish and naïve, but she is sophisticated enough to know the stork does not bring the baby. The condom may not be a perfect contraceptive, but it has the virtue of availability. For as little as 25 cents, a condom can be obtained in any drug store in the land, no questions asked. Condoms are even dispensed by vending machine in many localities. Therefore, it must be concluded from the tide of abortions, illegitimate births, and forced marriages that young people are not using even the condom. To supply them with a set of pills and instructions to start taking them on the fifth day of the cycle and continue for twenty days, then interrupt for ten days, and appear at the doctor's office twice a year for a checkup —and find the money to purchase the pills—to do all this and expect it to work with a girl who won't even insist that her partner use a condom is a little Pollyanaish. Viewed in this light, I don't believe that even if the Pill were made as easily available as aspirin that it would affect premarital pregnancy.

With the copulating teenager, we are dealing with factors far more complex than the simple joining of sperm and egg. When condoms are available and not being used, it is appropriate to ask, Why? I do not believe all pregnancies can be explained in terms of ignorance, accidents, or even foolishness. Psychologists have long pointed out that some girls want to become pregnant to punish their parents, the boy, and themselves for their guilt. Pregnancy is a means of escape from their home situation, the problems of career, or simply landing a boy they fear losing. I cannot conceive how a prescription for the Pill would combat these unconscious motivations for pregnancy any better than the condom.

The near future may alter this situation, however. A postcoital pill, taken at the end of a month in which copulation had occurred, would greatly change circumstances. The naïve, impulsive, or foolish girl who had sexual intercourse would then have the chance for sober reflection, a second chance for safety. It would make the problem of pregnancy control in young girls far easier for authorities—and VD control a possible calamity. That the postcoital pill would be an invitation to premarital sex is undeniable.

23. When Does Life Begin? Contraceptive or Abortifacient?

To my knowledge, no official legal, religious, or ethical objection exists anywhere in the world against family planning and contraception. The Roman Catholic Church, whose official views on contraception are among the most conservative, advocates family planning—by the rhythm method and sexual abstinence. Other major religions, including Protestant and Hebrew, have accepted the hormonal regulation of ovulation, as well as mechanical contraceptives such as condoms and diaphragms. Thus, the prevention of life has won worldwide endorsement.

The same may not be said for taking life. Murder of a living person is man's most heinous crime. Even such "justified" killing as occurs in self-defense, capital punishment, and war are now being criticized as immoral.

Nowhere has our attitude toward taking life been more rigid than in the issue of abortion. Our traditional view has been that the unborn fetus is the most innocent of beings and that taking that life is both morally wrong and legally a crime. Only a few nations (notably Japan) permit indiscriminate abortion. Until very recently, the only recognized legal justification for an abortion was to protect the health of the mother. Thus, the tragedy of the rape victim bearing an unwanted child could and did occur. During the last two years, campaigns have been launched in many states to liberalize abortion laws to permit the operation for specific indications. These are: (1) to protect the mental health of the mother; (2) when there is good reason to suspect that the baby may be deformed; (3) in victims of rape. A few states have passed such laws.

There is no issue of abortion in the use of the Pill as it is marketed today. No ovulation—no conception. Abortion cannot occur in the absence of conception, since life is not created. But the issue of abortion can indeed be raised concerning intrauterine devices and many of the contraceptive methods being projected for the near future. As a matter of fact, scientists are veering away from ovulation suppression in favor of "less drastic" methods.

But these advances in technique pose questions never before faced in this country. Abortion is usually considered to be a surgical procedure in which an implanted and growing fetus is destroyed or removed. The question being raised by many thoughtful men and women is this: Is the prevention of implantation an abortion? Stated another way: When does life really begin?

A review of the physiological processes leading to conception permits selection of several critical points at which it might be argued—and is indeed being argued—that life begins. The egg, released by the ovary, is picked up by the Fallopian tube, where it is surrounded and "attacked" by sperm, one of which penetrates and fertilizes the egg, joining the chromosomes of the father and mother. The fertilized egg then begins the process of cell division and growth. As this occurs, the fertilized egg (zygote) gradually descends the tube, arriving three days later in the cavity of the uterus. For three more days it floats in the cavity before attaching to and then implanting in the endometrium. Growth and development of the various tissues and body functions occur quite rapidly, and a heartbeat is customarily heard during the sixteenth week of pregnancy.

When in this process does a human life commence? It has been stated that life begins with contact between the egg and sperm;

when the sperm penetrates the egg and the chromosomes are united; when the first cell division occurs; when the egg implants in the uterus; and, since our legal definition of death is cessation of heartbeat, when the heart commences to beat in the sixteenth week.

Each of these possible times in the conceptual process has its proponents, each of whom vehemently insists that this is the beginning of life. For example, the late Dr. Carl Hartman, whose work in fertility control was of major importance, believed life began with the first cell division. Dr. John Rock states in his book *The Time Has Come*[48] that the Pill, as presently used, conforms to Catholic thinking, but considers "morning after" preparations to be abortifacients. Thus, to him life begins prior to implantation.

My own view parallels that of the American College of Obstetricians and Gynecologists and the Planned Parenthood-World Population Council. This concept accepts implantation of the fertilized egg as the beginning of life. The attachment of the fertilized egg to the endometrium is probably the most critical part of conception. It has been estimated that 15 to 20 per cent of fertilized eggs fail to implant and probably an equal number detach soon after implantation and are cast off with the menstrual flow. It seems reasonable to conclude that conception occurs when the process of implantation has been completed. But when is it completed? No specific answer is available, but purists insist that "completion" implies the establishment of maternal-fetal exchange.

Is the question of when life begins important? I believe it is. Our historic attitude toward abortion indicates that man cannot take human life casually. Our efforts to control population growth should not lead to mass guilt about methodology. It would be tragic if an effective postcoital pill or long-term progestational agent were declared illegal because of its abortifacient effect. One important legal factor should be mentioned, however. An abortion can occur only if conception occurs. Since there is no way of knowing, at such an early stage, whether conception has in fact occurred, an absolute diagnosis of abortion is similarly impossible.

This is not a problem of the future. It is a problem of today, since the available evidence suggests that the IUD works by preventing implantation of a fertilized ovum. But a person using the IUD never knows whether fertilization has occurred. This doubt might be a source of comfort to some individuals but an important concern to others. Anyone taking a long-term progestational agent that did not prevent ovulation would have to accept the fact that fertilization would inevitably occur, but not implantation.

The question of when life begins sounds like a problem for philosophers or theologians, but its importance cannot be discounted. Undoubtedly the problem is of little or no importance to many Pill takers or IUD users, but a more complete assessment of how these agents work should be made available to all concerned.

It seems to me that discussions of the question of when life begins must be started. Perhaps those religious organizations that specialize in ethical matters should reach a decision. Or perhaps this is a question to be decided in the hearts of men.

24. The Pill and the Catholic Church

THE CATHOLIC CHURCH is, and has been for a long time, receptive and responsive to all the valid arguments for a type of birth control properly known as child spacing. When ideally executed, it prevents the evil and danger of abortion. Spacing pregnancies strengthens the family, the functional and basic unit of society, since it permits parents to plan for the education and rearing of their children. Furthermore, control of pregnancy offers the only long-range hope for solutions to the world superpopulation problem and the ancillary spectre of world hunger.

The Church teaches that parents have the responsibility, before God, of deciding on the number of children they are able to rear and educate. But the Church does not believe that married couples have the inalienable right, before God, to choose among the existing birth control methods. It maintains that any agent, be it chemical or mechanical, that destroys or obstructs the male sperm or prevents the implantation of, or aborts, the fertilized ovum, is against the natural law. Therefore, the use of agents that affect these programs is immoral.

Prior to 1940, sexual continence was the only form of birth

control permitted by the Catholic Church. In that year, Pope Pius XII, in his encyclical *casti conubii* (Christian marriage), authorized Catholics to use the rhythm method. Thus, for those women who were blessed with regular ovulation and menstruation, an avenue was opened for the spacing of pregnancy. In this document, Pius XII repudiated Catholic concept dating from the thirteenth century that an infertile wife committed sin by continuing to have sexual relations with her husband. Prior to 1940, therefore, Catholic couples were permitted to have sexual intercourse only for the precise purpose of procreation. Any variation was sinful. A gynecologist, reflecting on this concept, might have had serious doubts about removal of the diseased uterus or tubes since, subsequent to this act, the female would sin with every act of intercourse.

The development of the oral contraceptive sent shock tremors through the entire Catholic system—the home, the parish church, the theologian's study, and the Papal chambers in Rome. The Pill seemed to catalyze the reaction concerning pregnancy control that had been smoldering in the church for many years. Actually, the catalyst was of such intensity that it ignited the flame of controversy.

Several factors were responsible. First, the Pill was not a mechanical device and, second, it had no connection with the sexual act. All previously used contraceptive devices intervened at the time of intercourse. The Pill did not. It simply used the same hormonal agents that the body uses during normal pregnancy to prevent further ovulation. This concept did not introduce a barrier since the male sperm were deposited in normal fashion and ascended the natural passages. The eggs developed in the ovary, even reached a certain position, but, as during pregnancy, the filmy capsule over the egg was not released. This was not abortion since, by definition, it is not possible to abort an unfertilized egg. One might rationalize that, instead of placing an artificial barrier in the female genital tract, the Pill simply prevented the dissolution of a natural barrier, the capsule, of the follicle containing the egg.

Ten years ago a Catholic patient and I were confronted with this problem somewhat prematurely. At that time I was using the basic ingredients of the Pill, although in slightly different formulation, to control abnormal uterine bleeding. This patient had a negative Rh blood factor and during six previous pregnancies had developed a rather high antibody titer. Although her last two babies had been born alive, both were born prematurely and survived only because of the ability of her pediatricians to perform exchange blood transfusions.

The patient elected not to have further pregnancies. I quite agreed with this decision and, if I had not been doing clinical investigation with the Pill, would have elected to do a vaginal hysterectomy and thus solve her abnormal bleeding problem. This avenue of approach is quite widely practiced by Catholic obstetricians and gynecologists since a definite disease process is being treated and, secondarily, pregnancy control is also accomplished. As a gynecologist, I consider this operative procedure superior to that of tubal ligation since the latter leaves behind a functionless uterus. But this functionless uterus is still subject to disease processes. Every year in our hospital we see two or three patients with cancer of the cervix or body of the uterus who previously had tubal ligation.

I told my patient that I could control her abnormal bleeding by the administration of the estrogen-progestin combination for twenty days of each month. As an added feature, it would also prevent ovulation and conception. Fortunately, my patient's brother was a professor of theology at a large Catholic university. I asked her to discuss this problem with him. The answer was immediate and direct. As long as I used the hormones for the control of bleeding, it was an acceptable procedure by the Catholic Church. The fact that ovulation did not occur was of no consequence. When I asked how I could utilize this method, I was told that this was a medical question and that the answer should be based on medical evidence. I elected to treat this patient for eleven of every twelve months, and I have done so successfully for the past ten years. Pregnancy has not occurred.

After the Pill was released and marketed for oral contraception and as knowledge increased about its method of action, it became difficult for many Catholic doctors, married couples, and theologians to comprehend a legitimate ban on this hormonal agent. The question was repeatedly asked, "Is the taking of the Pill an immoral act?" The usual answer was a statement issued by Pope Pius XII, who, on September 12, 1958, rejected as immoral the contraceptive use of drugs, pills, or medicines that "by preventing ovulation make fecundation impossible."

But this pronouncement did not solve the perplexity of the Catholic couple. Within the confines of Boston alone, two eminent Catholic gynecologists took exactly opposite viewpoints. Dr. John Rock has always insisted that the Pill is morally licit. He prescribes it freely for his Catholic patients and states with conviction, "The Pill is not immoral. Catholics can use the Pill, and should use it, with an easy conscience." Dr. William Lynch not only believes that the use of the Pill for pregnancy control violates Catholic teachings, he has described the Pill as "the most dangerous drug ever introduced for use by the healthy in respect to lethality and major complications."

Thus the door was opened to extensive debate and a torrent of spoken and written words from priests and laymen alike engulfed the Catholic couple. Professors and students of Catholic dogma suddenly became experts in the field of female reproductive physiology and discussed marital love with amazing frankness. Seldom in the history of the Church, which now claims a world membership of about half a billion people, has an issue produced such sharp and vocal division among its leaders. The Belgian Cardinal, Leon Joseph Suenens, declared before the Ecumenical Council in Rome, "We are faced with the problem, not because the Christian faithful are attempting to satisfy their passions and their egoism, but because the best among them are attempting with anguish to live a double loyalty to the Church's doctrines and to the needs of conjugal and parental love."

The resultant cleavage among the priests left millions of Catholic couples perplexed. Many made their own decisions and chose the Pill with or without a twinge of conscience or a confession.

One Catholic mother of four children put it succinctly, "The best time to be a Catholic is when you're very young or very old. In between, it's a problem. They say the Catholic Church is hard

254 Psychological, Social, and Moral Effects of the Pill

to live in and easy to die in and its true. But the pills, which so many in the Church are beginning to approve, will be a great help."[49]

This Catholic mother and her devout Catholic husband believed that they could not live in a state of grace and receive communion if they used ordinary contraceptives. These devices they regarded as sinful. "But for a thing to be a sin," she said, "three things are necessary: first, you must think it's a sin; second, it must be a grievous thing against God; and third, you must have done it voluntarily. Well, we don't think the pills are a sin, and our young priest said he saw nothing wrong with them either, so we don't confess using them, and we go to church and take communion. Young priests seem to be more understanding. In other parishes, the older priests do not give permission."

During the second session of Vatican Council II in 1963, the issue of the theology of marriage commanded the attention of the bishops. Then, in the spring of 1964, Pope Paul VI announced the formation of a Papal commission for the study of population, the family, and births. Many Catholics assumed that the Pope, having appointed such a deliberative body, gave ample evidence that the mind of the Church was open to the adoption of any new birth control method that was not unnatural. The character of the Commission fortified this assumption. Its sixty members, representing many countries, included theologians and prelates of high rank, doctors, scientists, sociologists, demographers, and married couples. In the spring of 1966, to broaden the basis of opinion, the Commission was enlarged by the addition of sixteen bishops, including several cardinals.

Because of the controversial aspect of the subject, members of the Commission were pledged to keep their deliberations secret from the press and the public. However, various unconfirmed leaks occurred and rumors were rampant. As these rumors were disseminated, many Catholics happily assumed that the Pill would eventually be accepted as legitimate. This was not an unreasonable assumption since it seemed unthinkable that the Pontiff would reject the conclusions reached by a majority of this commission. Furthermore, a number of prominent Catholic doctors, John Rock in the forefront, and scientists had been publicly insisting for some time that the Pill could be scientifically classed as a natural means of birth control. Some confessors argued that the Church was in a state of doubt, because of the reliably reported division of opinion within the Commission. Thus, the Pill was approved in some confessionals but not in others. As a matter of record, one Commission member was quoted in a discreet, sober report in the *Ladies' Home Journal,* "Of the 57 members of the Commission only about six are adamantly against birth control."

On June 28, 1966, the Commission submitted its eight hundred page report to the Pope. During the weeks of delay that followed, optimism was dominant. It was not until October 19, 1966, that the Pope revealed his interpretation of the report in an address to a group of Italian physicians. The conclusions of the Commission were not definitive, the Pope stated, and the need for supplementary study was evident. In the meantime, he declared, Catholics should give "faithful and generous observance to the Church's traditional teaching on artificial birth control." Reaction to the new postponement was instantaneous and at times somewhat derogatory. One eminent theologian remarked, "The Pope's position is ambivalent. He says he can't make up his mind on the subject. But he says he isn't in doubt." Somewhat ironically this student of the Church stated, "I do not know what to call this state of mind." An editorial in the *National Catholic Reporter* stated: "It is difficult indeed to find a meaningful distinction between a state of doubt and a 'moment of study and reflection.' It is still more difficult to understand how anyone can say he is not in a state of doubt on a given issue and yet be unable to speak his mind about it."

Reaction among the Catholic laity was for the most part critical. In some corners, Pope Paul was reproached for being indecisive; in others, his decision was called an act of cowardice. In others, he was flayed for his preoccupation with authority and obedience rather than with the welfare of most Catholics.

Other observers voiced approval of the Pope's decision, stating that he was using the delay to strengthen his support. But the Pope's uncertainty increased the anxiety of most Catholics. More and more they asked, "What shall we believe and whom can we trust?"

The dilemma of the Catholic laity was clearly expressed by one of its members, who questioned: "Whatever happened to the good old Catholic Church that could say this is right and that is wrong and not worry about contradicting itself? I miss that Church. What's going on?"

What is really going on is quite evident. Available information shows that in 1965, birth control was widely accepted and practiced in Catholic marriages. One poll suggested that between one-half and two-thirds of Catholics approved the use of contraceptives in marriage. A Gallup poll conducted in 1965 for the Population Council asked this question: "The Roman Catholic Church does not approve many methods of birth control. Do you believe that the Church should change its position on this matter?" Catholics answered affirmatively in higher numbers than non-Catholics. Fifty six per cent said yes, 22 per cent said no. The non-Catholic ratio was 53 per cent yes to 22 per cent no. The same survey asked if birth control information should be easily available to any single or married American woman. Catholics were 43 per cent in favor of giving it to single women, 81 per cent for giving it to married women.

At a recent seminar held at a Catholic university, the question of changing the current Church ruling on contraception was put to a group of marriage counselors, psychiatrists, doctors, social workers, theologians, and experts in church law. The response was overwhelmingly in favor of change, 63 to 3.

Another survey in 1967 of 1,800 women of childbearing age living in a county on Long Island was conducted. Two-thirds of the women in this survey were Catholic. The survey showed that 59.7 per cent of the Catholic wives between eighteen and forty-five were using birth control pills at the time or had within the last year. Of Catholic women going to mass each Sunday, 54.6 per cent were taking the Pill.

One of the most authoritative studies regarding the use of oral contraceptives by Catholic women was reported in 1966 by two sociologists, Professor Charles W. Westoff of Princeton University and Professor Norman D. Ryder of the University of Wisconsin. They stated that the proportion of Catholic wives complying with Catholic teachings on contraception was 70 per cent in 1955, 62 per cent in 1960, and by 1965 it had plunged to 47 per cent. Professor Westoff concluded: "The most significant finding of our study so far has been the increase in the use by married couples of fertility regulation in general and oral contraception in particular. This holds for non-Catholics and Catholics alike."

More compelling than these figures are the deeply human reasons given by those who have changed their minds on what methods of birth control are morally permissible. A nun in Milwaukee speaks out: "Because of the suffering I have personally observed among our Catholic people, my conviction is that the Church must do something!" Over and over, women refer to nervous breakdowns, alcoholism, the break-up of friends' marriages. Sally Cunneen, Associate Editor of the *Catholic Quarterly*, sent out questionnaires to Catholic women throughout the United States and published their responses in *Sex: Female; Religion: Catholic*.[50] She records a litany of experiences, the prime example of which sounds about like this: "We have eight children and find it impossible to give them the training and personal attention they deserve as individuals; I have had a nervous breakdown because of my frequent pregnancies." A Boston matron is quoted as saying, "There is widespread use of the Pill now, and in the majority of cases among young Catholic women. I think for valid reasons. No matter what the ultimate decision of the Pope, this will continue, even if it means disobedience and refusal of the sacraments." A Chicago wife complains: "In the area of sex, the Church preaches the rights of husbands to intercourse without any consideration of the wife. I sometimes get the feeling I'm property, not a person."

The geographic variation in acceptance of the Pill by American bishops was clearly shown in a decision made in January, 1967, by Archbishop Robert E. Lucey of San Antonio, Texas. At that time, Archbishop Lucey approved a community planned-parenthood proposal to establish twelve family-planning clinics under a grant from the United States Office of Economic Opportunity. Archbishop Lucey states, "Human beings should be judiciously in-

258 of the Pill

formed of scientific advances and exploration of methods by which spouses can be helped in arranging the numbers of their children." He continued: "In view of the inalienable right to marry and beget children, the question of how many children should be born belongs to the honest judgment of the parents."

Internal disputes are not unusual in Catholicism. However, it is questionable whether the extent of dissidence and critical independence recently exhibited would have occurred without the introduction of the contraceptive pill. The fact that these disagreements are being viewed by the general public is unusual.

Students of Catholic life have described a change. The familiar "stereotyped servility" of the layman and priest toward their superior in the clergy began to fade when substantial numbers of the laity developed equal or better education than their superiors. It was not sufficient for these individuals to pay homage, to obey obsolete rules on the basis of faith alone. The reverberating question "why" became dominant.

Catholic women are now cognizant of the fact that the Catholic Church is regrouping and revamping. These women are exercising their consciences in the matter of birth control with an autonomy few would have thought possible ten years ago. More Catholic women fear the physical effects, usually side effects of minor nature, of the Pill than fear eternal damnation. Most of these women have indicated that it would make little difference if the Vatican should announce a strong condemnation.

As another mother of two children explained, in response to Miss Cunneen's questionnaire, "The Church has no business in sexual matters. We, my husband and I, want to plan our family. We think birth control is reasonable. All this talk about violating a law of nature. What does that mean? Nobody can say for sure."[50]

On July 29, 1968, someone did say something for sure. On that day, Pope Paul VI issued his long-awaited encyclical, *Of Human Life*. That proclamation reaffirmed, in sweeping terms, the Church's historic stand against all "artificial" means of preventing childbirth. "Rome has spoken," runs an ancient proverb of the Roman Catholic Church, and, theoretically, the case is closed. But, apparently, in this case, the issue was far from closed. A deep and ominous rift was opened within the Church. The conservatives, including nearly all of the top hierarchy, stood firmly behind the Pope. But many priests and laymen rebelled openly.

Headlines in United States newspapers followed quickly: "Washington Priests Defy Cardinal on Birth Control," "Pope's Decision Viewed As Blow to Ecumenism," "Edict Called Not Infallible; Conscience Is Guide," "Pope Paul Challenged; Theologians Say His View on Birth Control Not Binding." Eight teachers at Boston College, four of them priests, criticized the encyclical, stating, "We feel that the recent Papal encyclical is not binding in conscience upon Catholics. Individual couples may at times find it desirable or even necessary to limit the size of their families, using the best means made available by medical science and consistent with the total value and dignity of human life."

The reactions of obstetricians in Boston to the Papal announcement ranged from dismay to total agreement, the latter view expressed by only one of a dozen physicians polled. "You can bet your life I'm pleased," exclaimed Dr. William A. Lynch, long an opponent of the Pill. "It's obvious that what the Pope is saying for Catholics is, 'This is it.'" Dr. Duncan E. Reid, Chairman of the Department of Obstetrics and Gynecology at Harvard Medical School, was one of those who registered displeasure with the Pope's statement. "I'm not surprised, however. The decision does not really affect the North American continent, where the Church probably has no great influence in the matter. I think that is a thing of the past, and we should not feel that this is disturbing," he said. Dr. Reid's concern was for less privileged nations of Latin America and Asia, where there was little evidence of birth control to begin with and where leadership would be apt, because of religious conviction, to do even less now that the Pope had spoken.

The Pope's stern "no," while not unexpected, is nonetheless a massive blow to liberals in the Church, to Catholics in general who entertained hope that Pope Paul would find a way at least to soften the Church's proscription. Many thought he would delegate authority for "individualization" to regional leaders or to parish priests. Some thought he would accept a pill that prevented ovulation but not one that produced an abortion.

The Papal encyclical is bound to have far-reaching effects. *Time* magazine stated in August, 1968: "It will almost certainly cause confusion and dissension in the Church, particularly among the young and now-disillusioned liberals, both clerics and laymen. Most important, it will inevitably increase doubts among many Catholics about their Church's ability to keep abreast of changing times."

Why did the Pope make the decision to condemn all means of birth control except rhythm? Why did Paul refuse to accept the majority opinion of his own commission? John Cardinal Heenan, the leader of Britain's 4 million Catholics and a member of the Papal commission, explains,

> The simple hope of Pope John that this intricate and delicate problem could be solved by a committee proved to be unfounded. Married couples were consulted, but their evidence was contradictory. Theologians disagreed, doctors disagreed. Needless to say, Cardinals also disagreed. The members of the Commission did not regard themselves as a jury. We did not think it was for us to pronounce the final verdict condemning or reprieving pills and other contraceptives. It was for us to give a view on the evidence before us. It was for the Pope alone to make the decision. It requires more heart-searching to give a final decision than to give an opinion.

Cardinal Heenan explained further:

> Should the Pope not have been guided by the opinions of the majority? In questions of ethics, it is not the number, but the weight of opinion that counts. Majority opinions are notoriously unreliable in moral issues. That is why a whole society can destroy itself. For example, the majority of Nazis decreed the sterilization of the unfit and the liquidation of the Jews. The Encyclical is gentle in tone. The Pope does not talk of sin or threaten damnation. He speaks with compassion because he knows the agony of those who are torn in conscience.

Cardinal Heenan concluded:

> Virginity has become a joke, and modesty is outmoded. Pills and condoms must be freely available to young students, schools must

teach boys and girls how to use contraceptives. Having large families—a form of delinquency—should be punished by law. This kind of doctrine is being preached in our country today. It helps you to see the Pope's point, doesn't it?

Despite the reasons *why* Pope Paul reached his decision, the encyclical has found little favor with the Catholic population of America, particularly those in their twenties. A recent Gallup poll[51] showed that only twenty-eight of every one hundred Catholics are in favor of Pope Paul's decision, fifty-four oppose and eighteen express no opinion. Almost 80 per cent of Catholics in their twenties disagreed with the decision. An editorial in *Life* magazine by John T. Elson is entitled: "The Tragic Error of Paul VI." Elson comments, "Pope Paul has shown little interest in diluting the power of his office and clearly has no desire to become Catholicism's first constitutional monarch. But in issuing his unenforceable decree on contraception, Paul has done damage to the prestige of the Papacy that may take him, and his successors, years to cure."

There is a bit more to the Pope's encyclical than a simple "no" to contraception. He declares that artificial birth control can lead to infidelity, immorality, loss of respect for women, even political dangers. These allegations brought this response from a woman in Malden, Massachusetts, in her letter to the Boston *Herald:* "Pope Paul contends that the use of so-called artificial contraceptives will lead to the eventual derogation of womanhood, because 'man may come to the point of considering her a mere instrument of enjoyment.' Doesn't he [the Pope] realize it is far more of a derogation for a husband to regard his wife as nothing more than a human Xerox machine, to be used only for the purpose of reproduction?"

The response par excellence of the user, the consumer, the buyer is expressed by this letter written by a Michigan mother to *Time* magazine:

> As a Catholic mother, wife, lover, therapist, chauffeur, social worker, comforter, healer, organizer, charity worker, cook, gardener, laundress, carpenter, secretary, messenger, nurse, artist, interior decorator, landscaper and homemaker, rhythm has wrought

babies, frustration, anger, frigidity, sorrow, incompatibility, bitch-
ery, unhappiness, disillusionment, dissatisfaction, discontent, bitter-
ness, instability and more babies.

To the Pill I can accredit harmony, communication, fulfillment,
satisfaction, happiness, stability, understanding, acceptance, relaxation, achievement, compatibility, courage, love, peace and
Christ.

The concern of the hierarchy of the Catholic Church was crystallized at the semiannual conference of 235 bishops of the U.S. held
in November, 1968. But even before the sessions started, almost
4,000 laymen demonstrated at the Mayflower Hotel in Washington, D.C. in support of 41 priests who had been set down by
Patrick Cardinal O'Boyle for their vocal denunciation of the
Pope's *Humanae Vitae*. In the Hilton Hotel, laymen milled through
the lobby chanting, "The Battle Hymn of the Republic" and "Impossible Dream." Whether these and other demonstrations affected
the decision of the bishops is unknown, but after numerous sessions
lasting well into the early morning hours, a pastoral letter was
composed and released. The bishops could not and did not contra-
dict the Papal edict but their decision made it clear that Catholics
in the U.S. who utilized contraceptive methods would not be
barred from the sacraments. While urging obedience to the concept set forth in *Humanae Vitae,* the bishops opened a small crevice
in the dam permitting Catholics to do exactly what they had been
told not to do. It was obvious that the bishops perceived an exodus
from the church of millions of Catholics who felt they could not
live in a state of sin.

The pastoral letter in essence stated, "No one following the
teaching of the church can deny the objective evil of contraception
itself. With pastoral solicitude we urge those who have resorted
to artificial contraception never to lose heart but to continue to
take full advantage of the strength which comes from the sacra-
ment of penance and the grace, healing, and peace in the Eucha-
rist."

Although the decision of the bishops apparently satisfied the
obvious and urgent need of many practicing Catholics, it did not
approach the edict of the bishops of France which urged couples

who, in their own conscience, felt the necessity to employ contraception for family planning, to do so. Another repudiation of Pope Paul's encyclical was formulated by Rev. Charles E. Curran and other theologians at the Catholic University of America. They stated that couples had the right to practice contraception if their consciences so dictated. As expressed by one spokesman for the assembled bishops, "No one can look into the heart and mind of an individual. He or she alone can do that. Having studied the variables, the advantages, the disadvantages, the individual alone can decide whether or not contraception is sinful."

Swiss theologian Hans Kung stated, "The encyclical is not an infallible teaching. I fear it creates a second Galileo case." As expressed, clearly and succinctly, by an American scholar in Rome, the problem of "Birth control is the Pope's Viet Nam."

The Pill and the Population Crisis

Every eight and one-half seconds a yellow light flashed on a machine during a recent meeting of the Population Association of America, reminding the members that another person was being born. Every minute the light flashed again, adding one immigrant to the population. Every twenty-three seconds it subtracted an emigrant, and a death was registered every seventeen seconds. The net increase in population added one person to the two million plus every fourteen and one-half seconds.

But the rate of population growth in the United States is at present relatively low, averaging just about 1 per cent per year. At this rate of increase, nonetheless, we may expect a doubling of our population in approximately seventy years. One can speculate on what this will mean in terms of the size of cities, housing, schools, medical services, recreational and cultural facilities.

For the United States the brake may be on. The birth rate, declining steadily since the late 1950's, headed still lower in 1968. It now appears that fewer than 3.5 million babies were born then. This is a decline of 200,000 from 1967, and the smallest number of births in any year since wartime 1945. Population experts, startled by the trend, are lopping millions off their projec-

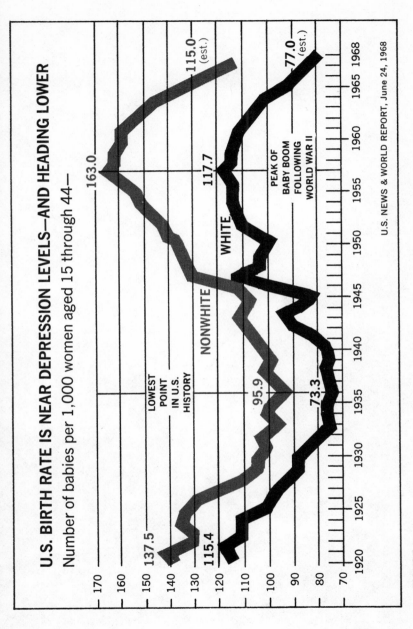

U.S. BIRTH RATE IS NEAR DEPRESSION LEVELS—AND HEADING LOWER

Number of babies per 1,000 women aged 15 through 44—

163.0

137.5

LOWEST
POINT
IN U.S.
HISTORY

NONWHITE

115.4

95.9

WHITE

117.7

73.3

115.0 (est.)

PEAK OF
BABY BOOM
FOLLOWING
WORLD WAR II

77.0 (est.)

1920 1925 1930 1935 1940 1945 1950 1955 1960 1965 1968

170 160 150 140 130 120 110 100 90 80 70

U.S. NEWS & WORLD REPORT, June 24, 1968

FIGURE I

tions for future years. The projected population of the United States by 1970 has been reduced from 212 million to 205 million. Businessmen, educators, and regional planners are scaling down long-range expansion.

Behind these major downward revisions in population growth is a drop in the birth rate in the United States that is now in its twelfth straight year, with no end in sight. Births hit a postwar peak of 123 births per 1,000 women, ages fifteen to forty-four, in 1957. The 1968 rate was probably down to eighty-two births per one thousand women, lowest since 1941 and close to the all-time low set in the Depression days of the 1930's. (See Chart on page 265.)

Why this decline? Officials in the U.S. Department of Health, Education and Welfare are frankly puzzled. They are unable to cite a single cause but list a number of contributing factors. One of the major factors is the pocketbook. Because of astronomical living costs, a large family can squeeze a budget dry. The cost of food, medical, and dental bills, larger homes and, perhaps most important, the cost of education tend to drop the curtain on family expansion.

Another factor is the attitude of churches suggesting the limitation of family size. Even the recent encyclical of Pope Paul listed four reasons why rhythm may be employed: social, medical, eugenic, and economic. Obviously any couple with a real problem can be easily covered by one of these indications.

There is no doubt that the Pill has played some role in the diminishing birth rate, but experts have pointed out that the decline began three years before the Pill was generally available, in 1957. Another factor may be the "uncertain outlook" for the future, the bomb, atomic annihilation. Many young adults wish to defer starting a family until their postgraduate education has been completed or they are established in business. Others prefer a sports car, a trip to Bermuda or Europe, a color TV, possibly even a mink coat. Pregnancy is planned for "next year" or perhaps "in a few years."

The working wife, replete with business image and check book, is frequently loathe to change the status quo. Children from large postwar families have grown up and many of these young adults are deciding that a smaller family is a better idea—perhaps only one or two children, so that "everyone will have it better."

While all of the factors listed are undoubtedly working in unison to reduce the birth rate, there is no doubt that the availability of the Pill and the IUD have greatly simplified the desired effect.

But despite the large growth of the last two decades, the United States, as a whole, remains rather sparsely populated by comparison with nations of Western Europe. According to *U.S. News and World Report*, America's population density per square mile (excluding Hawaii and Alaska) is 65 persons—against 934 in the Netherlands and 575 in Britain.[52] Two-thirds of the American people, however, are crowded into about 10 per cent of its land area (excluding Alaska). In the megalopolis now spreading from Boston to Washington, there are about 1,586 persons per square mile. And millions of people in these areas are finding life anything but an automated Garden of Eden. As crowded as New York City is now, if the present 2 per cent annual rate of world population growth continues, a population of 25 million crowded souls is predicted for that area alone. Obviously, something has to give. If golfers must get up at 4 A.M., and wait another four hours to tee off now, think what it will be like in the year 2000. That is, if there are any golf courses.

Today the population of the world is 3.5 billion, or nearly 1,000 times larger than it was 10,000 years ago.

Ansley J. Coale of Princeton University, President of the Population Association of America, recently commented, "If every woman in the United States were to experience the number of births she seems to want, the result would be an increase of 40 per cent per generation, or an average annual growth of more than 1 per cent. A continued growth at such a rate would be disastrous . . . leading to one person per square foot in 6 to 8 centuries." Coale prescribed an average, rather than a limit, of 2.3 children per couple. But Dr. William Lynch of Boston, head of the Catholic Rhythm Committee, does not believe the demographic experts. He comments, "Population prognostication, as well as other prognostication, has a history of remarkable error. After all, Solon in ancient Greece was advised that the world would starve to death or all people would be pushed off the edge of the world unless widespread abortion and contraception prevailed. None of these occurred. I believe a great deal of the writing in this regard has been in a panicky vein."

That was then and now is now, however. It took the United States 350 years to get to the 100 million population mark. It has taken just 52 years to get to the 200 million mark. It will take the United States as little as 30 years to get to the 300 million mark—unless something happens and, thanks to the Pill and the IUD, something is happening.

But what is happening elsewhere in the world? In Europe, the birth rate is even lower than in the United States, and declining steadily. Figures indicate that Catholic families, more and more, are practicing birth control. In Latin America, birth control has barely started catching on among the masses of people. Total population is growing at a rate of 3 per cent per year, highest in the world, in an area already struggling to provide the basic necessities for its people.

In France, a recent study showed about 56 per cent of practicing Catholics favored use of the Pill. And in Catholic Belgium, pharmacies report that the use of oral contraceptives is spreading over the entire country—despite the severity of penalties for any publicity given birth control. Latin America is the most dramatic symbol of lack of planning. It is in a race with the pace of history. It is making progress in the production of food and industrial and consumer goods, but its production of people is outrunning everything else. Its birth rate exceeds that of any other large area of the world, even surpassing Iindia's. It has a population of about 200 million now, which will be 300 million in the 1970's. Estimates for the year 2000 put its population at a staggering 600 to 700 million.

James Reston has noted that even the present population is beyond the control of even the best government in Latin America.[53] Almost two-thirds of the people are existing on 1,200 calories a day, less than half the U.S. average of 3,100. The per capita income is about $250 a year. Chile has the most liberal birth control policy in Latin America. It permits the distribution of birth control information and contraceptive devices. But poverty, religion, ignorance, and fear still create an almost unmanageable problem. It is illegal to have an abortion in Chile, but abortion is a flourishing business at $20 per operation; and for every 250,000 live births a year, there are 150,000 abortions. Even worse, the mortality rate of aborted mothers is fantastically high. Over 50 per cent of all maternal deaths are due to the complications of criminal abortion. Yet the annual population growth of 2.4 per cent is running well ahead of the 1.9 per cent growth of food production.

When the growth rate of a population is 2.5 per cent annually, it doubles in twenty-eight years. When the rate of increase is 3.5 per cent annually, the doubling time is reduced to twenty years. Such shortening periods for doubling hardly provide the opportunity for adaptation or change of direction.

At the time of Christ, the world contained some 250 million people and it took 1,650 years for this to double. The next doubling period was shortened to 200 years, so that the world population in 1850 numbered 1 billion. Seventy-five years later, in 1925, a population of 2 billion was reached. On January 1, 1968, the world population was 3.4 billion and the estimate for 1980 is 4 billion, for 1990 5 billion, and for the year 2000, assuming constant trends, 6.5 billion.

Dr. John Maier, Associate Director for the Medical and National Sciences of the Rockefeller Foundation, reminds us that population trends can be reversed but that the problems are multiple and complex. As Dr. Maier notes, "Reduction of the rate of population growth is not a sufficient condition for social and economic development. Other means, such as industrialization, must proceed along with such reduction. But it is clear that it is a necessary condition without which the development process is seriously handicapped."

There are available methods for improving world agriculture. And the methods for family planning by contraceptive techniques have been broadened in recent years. The essential need is rapid use of both measures throughout the world.

What is being done in the so-called "under-privileged" countries? The population of India, now 525 million, is increasing at the rate of 1 million a month. James Lelyveld, writing in *The New York Times,* has reported the progress since 1965.[54] Three years ago, the intrauterine device was given an extensive trial in preference to the Pill for two major reasons: First, India's family-planning program effectively reached only about 5 per cent of the nation's million fertile couples. Those accepting the Pill had a much higher level of literacy than the ordinary Indian. Second, it was impossible to provide the necessary follow-up examinations of women taking the Pill. But a large proportion of Indian women who tried the IUD complained of pain and profuse bleeding. So the search began for a better method. In 1967, sterilization of the male was initiated, aided and abetted by a bonus of a transistor radio given to each applicant. In one year almost two million male sterilizations were done and family planners were optimistic. But subsequent figures indicated that this procedure had no great effect on the birth rate. The major reason was that most of those who were willing to undergo the operation already had four or five children, instead of the two or three urged by the Government.

At the request of the Ford Foundation, a team of experts from the Arthur D. Little Company of Cambridge, Massachusetts, a top-notch industrial research organization, began an in-depth study of the problem. As a result of their recommendations, the condom is about to receive the biggest promotional drive ever given any new product in India. On October 1, 1968, over 80,000 small retail outlets throughout the country were stocked with condoms and featured huge posters in twelve languages stating: "Men! The Power To Prevent Birth Is In Your Hands. Use Nirodhs For Family Planning." Nirodh is the Hindu word for "prevention" and the condoms will be sold for less than a penny each.

A marketing scheme, suggested by the Arthur D. Little Company, coordinates major private corporations with experience in the Indian marketplace. A cigarette maker, Imperial Tobacco, a soap maker, Hindustan Lever, a battery maker, Union Carbide, and two tea companies, Lipton and Brooke Bond, have joined forces under the aegis of the Family Planning Ministry. Their 500,000 regular outlets will be available for the distribution and sale of condoms. Although the program will guarantee only marginal profit to the companies, their incentive is said to be experience in what the experts call "demand creation." This has boiled down to a hard-sell program, and as one marketing expert stated, "This is one program that won't be run by a lady gynecologist and a bunch of social workers."

In Russia, medical researchers are conducting tests of modern contraceptive agents including the Pill despite a background of official frowns. I vividly remember my Intourist guide looking at the structural formula of one of my slides during my check-in at the air terminal in Moscow. This episode occurred in 1963 during a meeting of the International Cancer Conference. Although the slide carried no identifying label, the guide, obviously cognizant of my work, exclaimed, "But, Dr. Kistner, isn't this the formula for Enovid, the oral contraceptive? This conference is on cancer, not family planning." I had difficulty in explaining to this brilliant young man that my paper was on the effects of progestins, like Enovid, on pre-malignant and malignant changes in the uterine lining.

Russians have a great desire for large families and for children, but most city dwellers hold jobs and the newer housing projects offer little welcome to more than one, possibly two, children. As a result some of the older technics still being used require that a woman soak for a few hours in a hot bath generously sprinkled with dry mustard or drink a potion containing quinine or coconut oil. Some of the younger Russians have been told that pregnancy may be avoided by avoiding simultaneous climax. *New York Times* correspondent Raymond H. Anderson states that "many a crisis in university dormitories has resulted from this belief."

Other up-to-date methods are available and the intrauterine device has recently been given the blessing of Soviet health leaders. More than 300,000 IUD's have already been produced in the Soviet Union and the total output in 1969 will reach one million. Among the Soviet Union's population of 230 million are about 55 million women of child-bearing age. Diaphragms are unpopular because the woman must make frequent clinic visits for check-up. Soviet-made condoms may be purchased for about two cents each but the quality is poor and has led to numerous "shotgun" weddings. For married couples who enjoy Russian roulette, the Russian condom provides the same aura of expectancy.

The general dissatisfaction with present family planning methods is reflected by the crowds at assembly-line abortion clinics. During the early days of Bolshevik emancipation of women, in 1920, abortions were legalized. During the war years, however, beginning about 1936, they were prohibited. But even prison terms did not suppress illegal abortions and, in 1955, abortions were again permitted "upon request." The cost of an abortion in Moscow is $5.50 but the conditions under which they are performed are less than ideal.

Raymond Anderson has vividly described the scene: "Girls of 17 may find themselves waiting amid callous, middle-aged women, with half a dozen abortions behind them, in a crowded room with operations being performed three at a time in an atmosphere as impersonal as a supermarket checkout counter. Anesthesia is not used and the screams of pain are unnerving to those waiting their turn." After five or six abortions a woman may finally decide that she desires a child. Too late. Either the lining of the womb has been excessively scarred or the tubes are closed from previous post-abortal infection. But Soviet women still frequent the clinics out of desperation. According to Anderson, the women fear and dislike abortions and they will be happy to see the clinics padlocked as soon as the IUD appears on the market. Research on the Pill continues in Russia, and limited clinical trials are being carried out. The Soviets are reportedly tooling up for production of an estrogen-progestin similar to U.S. brands. The selection of the IUD over the Pill is looked upon as a political move by Dr. Louis Hellman. He stated, "I think it would have been a diplomatic setback for the Russians to copy a European method, since the Pill is so intimately associated with the Free World." Dr. William Inman, senior medical officer of the Committee on Drug Safety in London, stated, "The Russians are not world leaders in the manufacture of pharmaceuticals so it may be easier for them to concentrate on IUD's, which happen to cost less."

This desire is not shared by Soviet leaders, however. They

would like to see more babies, not fewer. The birth rate has fallen from 44 per 1,000 in 1926 to only 18 per 1,000 in 1966. As an incentive to procreation, all employed men over 18 and working married women without children pay a 7 per cent "childlessness" tax. But the hard-working Russian woman is rebellious and my bet is that the Pill, or a Soviet innovation, will soon be available.

What can be accomplished in an "under-developed" country has been demonstrated in Malaysia. The birth rate in that country declined from 46.2 in 1957 to 37.3 in 1966 even before a well-planned Government program was started. This was attributed to: (1) a rise in the average age of marriage, (2) efforts of the voluntary family-planning association, (3) commercial sales of oral contraceptives, (4) birth control prescribed by private physicians, and (5) abortion.

Although abortion is illegal except to save a woman's life, nearly one-half of the admissions to the General Hospital of Kuala Lumpur Department of Gynecology are for evacuation of the uterus following attempted abortion. In the General Hospital of Alor Star, the capital of the State of Kedah, with three thousand deliveries a year, five hundred women are admitted annually suffering from the effects of abortion, many of them suspected of being induced.

The main method of contraception used is that of oral contraceptives, sold at the price of one Malaysian dollar (33 U.S. cents) per month, with free dispensing to those unable to pay. The intrauterine device, inserted for only 5 per cent of women accepting family planning, is available at a nominal charge.

A striking accomplishment of the program in Malaysia is that it is reaching the younger, more fertile groups because initial efforts are concentrated in the maternity hospitals during the postpartum period, when women are most receptive to the idea of family planning. Oral contraceptives are started immediately after the completion of an abortion and shortly after delivery since it has been shown of women who become pregnant after delivery, one-half conceive within three months, and four-fifths within one year.

Malaysian family-planning leaders had the foresight in 1967 to conduct a national survey that showed that 31 per cent of the married women in the metropolitan areas and 2 per cent of rural women were using contraception. The Malaysian government had appropriated $200,000 to the ongoing program, and Sweden is contributing contraceptive materials and vehicles. The Ford Foundation has awarded a two-year grant of $120,000 (Malaysian) for training, evaluation, and equipment. The National Family Planning Program of Malaysia faces a number of problems but they are organized, determined, and undoubtedly will succeed.

Unless individuals and family-planning organizations are able to control the growth rate of population, nations may be forced to take over. "If the birth rate can't be controlled by voluntary means, then it is, I believe, a necessary and proper function of the government to take steps to reduce it," writes Dr. Melvin M. Ketchel, a Professor of Physiology at Tufts School of Medicine in Boston.[55] Dr. Ketchel suggested that drugs be developed to control fertility in the whole population; drugs that could, for example, be administered to urban centers through the water supply. This is not unlike the suggestion that I made in an earlier chapter whereby all human females would be infertile unless a specific medication was taken to make them fertile. However salutary a method of this type might be, Dr. Ketchel proposed a set of characteristics for the agent which, at least for the moment, seem unlikely from a practical standpoint. He suggested that such an agent should: (1) lend itself easily to the intake of everyone—such as in the water supply; (2) be harmless with no danger to health or to the development of fetuses or children; (3) be inexpensive; (4) have a reversible effect; (5) have an antidote; that is, it should not interfere with the family planning of individual couples; and (6) have no effect on the sexual activity of the individuals in the population. If anyone knows of a compound with these utopian propensities, please call me.

Meanwhile, back at the ranch in the United States, what progress has been made to provide assistance to those who need it most? Recent studies of fertility rates in the United States have shown the rate to be highest in those areas with the lowest per capita income. The lowest birth rate occurs in families whose an-

276 Psychological, Social, and Moral Effects of the Pill

nual income is between $5,000 and $15,000. High birth rates are found in families whose income is either below $5,000 or above $15,000. In the latter group it is desirable, in the former it is deplorable. The motivation to control family size is notoriously poor in the lower-income group, and this is emphasized in areas where welfare payments actually benefit the unmarried mother of numerous children. The deprived American Negro has, in many instances, resisted assistance in the field of family planning both for this reason and a sense of stifling of racial growth.

But progress is being made. Health-department family-planning programs can be, and are, financed through a variety of sources: federal, state, county, or city, usually in some combination. The interest of the federal government has been made clear by the policies and programs of the relevant federal agencies. In January, 1966, Secretary of Health, Education and Welfare John Gardner issued the first departmental policy on family planning and assigned overall responsibility to Assistant Secretary Philip R. Lee, M.D. It has been estimated that in 1966, $3 million were utilized to finance family-planning services.[56][57]

To date, federal support for health-department family-planning programs has been channeled mainly through the state formula grants for Maternal and Child Health and through the more recent program of project grants for Maternal and Infant Care. For both public and voluntary agencies, a more direct and accessible source of federal support to initiate or expand family planning has been the Community Action Program of the Office of Economic Opportunity and, to date, at least sixteen health departments have secured these grants together with thirty-nine other agencies. Undoubtedly many more will follow.[58][59]

Congress has recently enacted a new and most promising source of additional financial support: *The Comprehensive Health Planning and Public Health Services Amendments* (Senate-3008; House of Representatives-18231). In testimony on this legislation, Dr. Philip R. Lee stated, "We do not have adequate funds to support it. We estimate that we will need at least $15 million next year to support requests that we are presently expecting, and that more will be needed in subsequent years."

Undersecretary Cohen's letter to the House Committee stated, "For the purpose of supporting programs in the field of family planning, our present plans contemplate $20 million in fiscal year 1968, $25 million in fiscal year 1969, and $30 million in fiscal year 1970."

On the other hand, the Office of Economic Opportunity estimated the cost of a five-year program at 126 million dollars. This estimate is based on their assumption that only one-half of the women will accept services and that only 40 per cent of those will effectively practice birth control. Practically speaking, however, the total budget for population problems in fiscal 1967 was just a little over 25 million dollars and, of this, two-thirds was earmarked for assistance abroad, research, and training.

There is no doubt that the war in Vietnam has diminished the expansion plan of the government for family-planning services.[43] The Planned Parenthood-World Population group surveyed fifty-four antipoverty birth control programs in 1967 and noted that sixteen would have to be disbanded for lack of government funds. An attempt was made to divert 24 million dollars from the United States Public Health Service to bridge this deficit. However, this also failed because of lack of funds.

It has become evident that government funds must be specifically earmarked for birth control services to the indigent in order to establish such agencies on a firm basis. An attempt was made to do just this in 1966 when Senator Joseph B. Tydings of Maryland proposed that the government specify 15 million dollars for birth control services in fiscal 1968, increasing this by 15 million dollars yearly to a maintenance allocation of 75 million dollars yearly. But Senator Tydings was informed by Undersecretary of Health, Education and Welfare Wilbur J. Cohen that public-health funds in the amount of 20 million dollars would be available for family planning under the comprehensive Health Services Act of 1966. Apparently this would have evolved if Congress had voted a large increase for all health services, but it did not. Since the states either had to divert funds from existing programs into birth control or neglect birth control completely, the effect was obvious. In the same fashion, the Office of Economic Opportunity

278 Psychological, Social, and Moral Effects of the Pill

did not specifically diminish budgets for birth control programs. The cutback was in the community-action program and, since birth control programs derive their funds from the community-action budget, the local communities reacted as expected. More funds were directed to politically popular programs, and family planning suffered.

Thus there are two major administrative difficulties delaying the effectiveness of a proven program. At the grass-roots level, the family planners have stated that the government must clearly earmark funds for their program. But officials at the Office of Economic Opportunity and at Health, Education and Welfare believe that the states and the community should divide their allocation according to their own priority and decision.

Another major problem exists in Washington. In an effort to properly pigeonhole birth control, Dr. Phillip Lee of Health, Education and Welfare has stated that family planning is more a health than a welfare program and should be shifted from the welfare-oriented Children's Bureau to Public Health. But neither the Children's Bureau nor the Public Health Department is anxious for a change.

It seems quite obvious to all that the answer to ending poverty in the United States is not as simple as government subsidization of Planned-Parenthood clinics. This will not provide additional jobs, on-the-job training, better housing or more food. But the opportunity for child spacing will have its major effect upon the child. Better education, closer parental guidance and mental stimulation will assist his escape from the poverty cycle.

The problem in the United States, therefore, seems solvable and depends upon clear-cut organization and funding in Washington. In the large metropolitan areas advantage should be taken of the teaching hospitals and their large resident and intern staffs. In many areas, Medicaid will solve the financial difficulty. Community action is obviously necessary to halt the constant stifling of hope and deteriorating health of women who, in the estimation of Margaret Sanger, founder of the Planned Parenthood movement, envision themselves as "pregnant year after year like so many automatic breeding machines."

Thus, we are just beginning our major effort to place the creation of life under the guidance of man's ethic and intellect. It appears as a well-timed measure since the rate of population growth is the single most important obstacle to economic and social development in underdeveloped countries. According to Dr. Lauchlin Currie, head of the Department of Economics at the National University of Colombia, population growth outranks even the threat of nuclear warfare. Dr. Currie points out that efforts to decrease birth rates among those who most need family planning have not been effective. The poor, and particularly the rural poor, are the most difficult to reach and influence.

Dr. Currie insists that a strong effort must be made to bring about a rapid rise in the economic and educational levels of the poorest half of the population in order to secure a "breakthrough" in the vicious circle of poverty, ignorance, high birth rate, etc. His conclusion: Both family planning and economic and social planning should be effected at the same time.

On Human Rights Day in December, 1967, at the United Nations, thirty world leaders, representing many political and religious beliefs, countries large and small, highly developed and lesser-developed, signed a joint statement. This declaration is as follows:

STATEMENT ON POPULATION
BY WORLD LEADERS

The peace of the world is of paramount importance to the community of nations, and our governments are devoting their best efforts to improving the prospects for peace in this and succeeding generations. But another great problem threatens the world—a problem less visible but no less immediate. That is the problem of unplanned population growth.

It took mankind all of recorded time until the middle of the last century to achieve a population of one billion. Yet it took less than a hundred years to add the second billion, and only thirty years to add the third. At today's rate of increase, there will be four billion people by 1975 and nearly seven billion by the year 2000. This unprecedented increase presents us with a situation unique in human affairs and a problem that grows more urgent with each passing day.

The numbers themselves are striking, but their implications are of far greater significance. Too rapid population growth seriously hampers efforts to raise living standards, to further education, to improve health and sanitation, to provide better housing and transportation, to forward cultural and recreational opportunities—and even in some countries to assure sufficient food. In short, the human aspiration, common to men everywhere, to live a better life is being frustrated and jeopardized.

As heads of governments actively concerned with the population problem, we share these convictions:

We believe that the population problem must be recognized as a principal element in long-range national planning if governments are to achieve their economic goals and fulfill the aspirations of their people.

We believe that the great majority of parents desire to have the knowledge and the means to plan their families; that the opportunity to decide the number and spacing of children is a basic human right.

We believe that lasting and meaningful peace will depend to a considerable measure upon how the challenge of population growth is met.

We believe that the objective of family planning is the enrichment of human life, not its restriction; that family planning, by assuring greater opportunity to each person, frees man to attain his individual dignity and reach his full potential.

Recognizing that family planning is in the vital interest of both the nation and the family, we, the undersigned, earnestly hope that leaders around the world will share our views and join with us in this great challenge for the well-being and happiness of people everywhere.

HAROLD HOLT
Prime Minister of Australia

DR. CARLOS LLERAS RESTREPO
President of Colombia

ERROL W. BARROW
Prime Minister of Barbados

JENS OTTO KRAG
Prime Minister of Denmark

DR. JOAQUIN BALAGUER
President of Dominican Republic

PER BORTEN
Prime Minister of Norway

DR. URHO KEKKONEN
President of Finland

LT. GEN. J. A. ANKRAH
*Chairman of the
National Liberation Council
of Ghana*

MME. INDIRA GANDHI
Prime Minister of India

GENERAL SUHARTO
Acting President of Indonesia

SHAH MOHAMMAD REZA PAHLAVI
Emperor of Iran

EISAKO SATO
Prime Minister of Japan

HIS MAJESTY HUSSEIN
*King of Hashemite Kingdom
of Jordan*

GENERAL CHUNG HEE PARK
President of Republic of Korea

TUNKU ABDUL RAHMAN
Prime Minister of Malaysia

HIS MAJESTY HASSAN II
King of Morocco

HIS MAJESTY MAHENDRA
King of Nepal

DR. J. ZIJLSTRA
Prime Minister of The Netherlands

KEITH HOLYOAKE
Prime Minister of New Zealand

FIELD MARSHAL MOHAMMED
AYUB KHAN
President of Pakistan

FERDINAND E. MARCOS
*President of Republic
of the Philippines*

LEE KWAN YEW
Prime Minister of Singapore

TAGE ERLANDER
Prime Minister of Sweden

THANOM KITTIKACHORN
Prime Minister of Thailand

ERIC WILLIAMS
*Prime Minister of Trinidad
and Tobago*

HABIB BOURGUIBA
President of Tunisia

GAMAL ABDEL NASSER
President of UAR

HAROLD WILSON
Prime Minister of United Kingdom

LYNDON B. JOHNSON
*President of United States
of America*

MARSHAL JOSIP BROZ-TITO
President of Yugoslavia

Questions Women Ask Most About "The Pill"

D URING THE LAST seven years I have spoken frequently before audiences made up chiefly of women taking the Pill. During this time I have accumulated several hundred questions asked most frequently. Essentially, the questions are the same as those asked by my patients, either in my office or on the telephone. This selection is offered as a quick reference guide should problems and misapprehensions arise. It will save both you and your doctor valuable time if you are acquainted with the information contained in the answers I give to these most frequently asked questions.

Q. *How many varieties of the pill are now available?*

A. At the present time there are 20 varieties of the Pill (actually a tablet since pills are spherical) on the market in the United States which may be used for conception control. The majority of these are *combinations* of female hormones, *estrogen* and *progestin,* very similar to the natural secretions of the ovary. The sequential pills employ an estrogen for fourteen to sixteen days followed by combination for the last five days. There are slight variations in the pills that are of importance in selection for different individuals. (See Table II on p. 51.)

Q. *Must the pills be taken under a physician's care?*

A. Yes. Because this is so, it is not only inadvisable, it is danger-ous to give your pills to someone else to take.

Q. *Will I continue to have menstrual periods while using the oral method of contraception?*

A. Yes—except that your cycles are likely to be more regular and your flow somewhat lighter. Occasionally there may be no flow at all, but this is of no significance. If you now suffer from menstrual pain or premenstrual tension, it is a good bet that the Pill will reduce or eliminate these discomforts.

Q. *Do I take the pills every day of the month?*

A. No, oral contraceptives are taken for regular periods of time, in sequence, usually twenty or twenty-one days during each men-strual cycle. If your doctor has prescribed some of the newer agents combining several ingredients you will take a pill every day, but they may be of varying strengths or seven of them may be only "dummy" pills. For example, in one preparation on the market a pill containing estrogen and progestin is taken for twenty-one days. Then the next seven pills are "dummies," placed in se-quence in the package so that a pill is taken every day for four weeks. This is merely a method of simplifying pill taking. Then, two or three days after the "hormone" pill is discontinued, a normal bleeding episode occurs. This continues for another two or three days while the dummies are taken. Another pill, not yet marketed, mimics the hormonal changes during the normal menstrual cycle by gradually increasing the amount of estrogen for twenty-one days—then the last seven pills contain both an estrogen and a progestin. After the last combined pill is taken, the cycle is re-started with a *low dose* estrogen pill. Because of sudden drop in hormones, a period—really a "withdrawal flow"—then occurs.

Q. *What is the best time of day to take the Pill?*

A. It really makes no difference as long as a regular habit is formed. When starting patients on the Pill I tell them to take it with the evening meal, since I believe this will diminish the inci-dence of nausea.

Q. *Can I get pregnant if I forget just one pill during the 20- or 21-day program?*

A. The chances are slight, but skipping even one pill *can* result in pregnancy. This is even more plausible when one is taking the sequential-type pills, rather than the combined variety. However, it is important for you to take the Pill every day for twenty or twenty-one days without fail. The risk of pregnancy increases with each pill missed; thus, if you should skip a day, it is all the more important to continue the pills for the remainder of the 20- or 21-day program. I usually tell my patients to take the "skipped" pill the next morning and to follow through with the regular pill that night.

Q. *If I missed taking my pills for two consecutive days, should I then take three pills the third day?*

A. No, I think it would be adequate to take one pill in the morning and one pill in the evening on the day on which you re-start and then keep up with one pill daily for the completion of the 20- or 21-day cycle. Again, the risk of pregnancy increases with each pill missed.

Q. *If I miss a pill, should I use another form of contraception during the rest of that cycle?*

A. It's a good idea. By employing another method of birth control, you will be doubly protected against pregnancy unless, of course, you ovulated within the first twenty-four hours after missing one pill. Most of the time, however, ovulation occurs very early in the pill-taking cycle, particularly if there has been a delay in starting a new cycle. I always advise my patients to refrain from intercourse during the first seven days of the *first* cycle of pill treatment.

Q. *Exactly how do the pills prevent conception?*

A. The principal action of the pills is to stop the monthly release of an egg. However, this is not the only reason pills are effective. Some physicians feel that a part of the action of the pill is to change the lining of the womb so that it is difficult for an egg to implant. Other physicians feel that still another action of the pills might contribute to their effectiveness—their effect on cervical mucus. This prevents the penetration of sperm through the cervix. Still another effect is possible. This concerns the rate of transport of the egg through the tube into the lining of the womb. If the egg arrives in the uterus *too early or too late,* it will not implant.

The lining of the womb is stimulated to grow each month by the action of estrogen for the first fourteen days, then becomes ideally developed for implantation by the action of estrogen and progesterone (from the ovary) after ovulation. In order for the egg to implant and grow, the lining of the womb must be just right and this occurs about six days after ovulation. If the egg arrives in the uterus too soon, the lining will not accept it; if it arrives too late, degenerative changes have already occurred in the lining and this, too, prevents normal implantation.

Q. *While using the Pill, will I have my menstrual periods?*

A. Yes—except that your cycles are likely to be more regular and your flow somewhat lighter. Your periods will begin usually within two to three days after you've taken the last (twentieth or twenty-first) pill in each month's program. In some patients it occurs sooner, in others later. Some patients have no flow at all, and this is simply due to the fact that the lining of the womb has not built up sufficiently during the twenty or twenty-one days. This is of no significance and you should restart the pills five days after the last pill in the previous cycle has been taken. If you now suffer from menstrual pain or premenstrual tension, it is a good bet that the Pill will reduce or eliminate these discomforts.

Q. *Can an overdose of pills be harmful?*

A. No ill effects have been reported from an overdose of oral contraceptives—and that includes several accidents in which children swallowed over twenty pills at one time!

Q. *How soon after I've had a baby can I start on the Pill?*

A. Your doctor will advise you in this regard. Most gynecologists and obstetricians start a patient on the Pill after she has had her first spontaneous menstrual period after delivery. However, if the patient has not had a period by the time of the six-week check-up following delivery, many physicians will initiate therapy at that time. Some physicians, particularly in large metropolitan hospitals, give the Pill as soon as the patient leaves the hospital. The reason for this is simple. Many of these women become pregnant before they return for their six-week check-up.

Q. *Can I nurse my baby while using the pills?*

A. Your doctor will decide this. He may tell you not to take the pills until after you have finished the nursing period, or he may allow you to start the new low-dosage pills five to eight weeks after delivery. In part, your doctor's decision will be based on your body's ability to produce enough milk for your baby.

Q. *What should I do if I have breakthrough bleeding while taking the Pill?*

A. There are two ways of handling this problem. First, if the bleeding occurs after the seventeenth or eighteenth pill and it is rather profuse, you may stop taking the pills at this time and permit the flow to occur, starting the next cycle of pills five days from the start of flow. If spotting or light bleeding occurs about the thirteenth or fourteenth pill, I usually tell my patients to double the dose for the remainder of that cycle and then start anew during the next cycle with the regular one-pill-a-day routine. In most instances, spotting and bleeding will disappear by the third or fourth cycle of pills.

Q. *Doesn't the body build up poisons in the blood if a normal menstrual flow does not occur after taking the Pill?*

A. No, the menstrual flow has absolutely nothing to do with getting rid of poisonous wastes in the body. This is handled by the kidneys and by the intestinal tract. The flow that occurs normally is simply the result of not getting pregnant. Menstruation merely permits the lining of the womb, which is built up to receive the fertilized egg, to degenerate and escape. Therefore, if you have a very scanty flow after taking the Pill, disregard it.

Q. *What would happen if I took the pill continuously even after the twenty or twenty-one days?*

A. Nothing, except you would not have a period until you did stop the Pill. I have treated patients for certain diseases, such as endometriosis (Endometriosis is a growth of tissues on the tubes, ovaries, bowel, and bladder that is exactly the same as that which lines the uterus. The lining of the womb is called the "endometrium"; when tissue like endometrium grows inside the body cavity it is called "endometriosis.") by having them take the Pill continuously for as long as two years and during this time they had no menstrual periods. Usually after thirty-five or forty days "breakthrough bleeding" will occur. It is then necessary to double the dose. However, if you wish to delay a bleeding episode for a week or two weeks, or even for two months, no harm will result. Many athletes and actresses do exactly this if they do not wish to menstruate at a certain time.

Q. *In the sequential pills, why are there fourteen white and five colored pills and what do the colored pills do that the white ones do not?*

A. In the sequential treatment method, the first fourteen pills in Ortho-Novum and Norquen are estrogen. In C-Quens the first fifteen and in Oracon the first sixteen pills are estrogen. The next five pills are a combination of estrogen and a progestin, exactly the same as in most of the other combined pills. The combination pills, the last five in the cycle, change the lining of the womb so that a more uniform and more normal flow is obtained. Suppression of ovulation and prevention of pregnancy can be obtained by use of estrogen alone, if given in adequate amount. However, when this was tried many years ago, the resulting flow was occasionally profuse and sometimes irregular.

Q. *Is it possible to change from one brand of pill to another safely? For example, from Enovid to Ortho-Novum?*

A. Yes, it is possible to change. However, I would warn you that whenever you shift from one brand to another you must refrain from intercourse during the first seven days of the first cycle with the new pill. This is particularly true if the newer pill contains a lesser amount of estrogen. It would be quite simple for the pituitary gland to release the necessary hormones to cause ovulation if you shifted to a pill containing only one half of the estrogen in the previous pill.

Q. *My husband is away on temporary duty with the Air Force and I have stopped taking the Pill. When should I start taking it again before he gets back?*

A. I would advise that you have one full cycle of pill taking with one withdrawal flow before he returns.

Q. *You mentioned that there are different kinds of pills. Is there a reason for one doctor to give a different pill to every patient?*

A. Well, I would not say that every patient should get a different type of pill, but it is certainly true that some patients respond better, with less side effects, to one type of pill than another. This is something that your own physician will determine and it is fortunate that, at the present time, we now have twenty different combinations of pills from which to make a selection.

Q. *If I stop taking the Pill for six months and decide to start again, how long should I take them before having intercourse?*

A. I would suggest that you refrain from intercourse for the first seven days after starting the pills anew. It is just possible you might ovulate early during this cycle and there would be insufficient time for the Pill to have its full effect.

Q. *If no menstrual flow occurs after taking the pill for twenty or twenty-one days, how do I know when to start the pill?*

A. Always start five days after the twentieth pill of the last cycle.

Q. *If I am nursing my baby and no menstruation occurs, how do I know when to start the pill?*

A. Your physician will decide this, but you do not have to await a menstrual flow. You simply start taking the pills for twenty days and then the withdrawal flow will occur. You then start a regular sequence.

Q. *Could a girl of twelve or thirteen years of age be given the Pill daily and constantly to prevent her from suffering through menstrual periods each month?*

A. If the child had already acquired full growth stature, and I assume that she would if she were ovulating and menstruating regularly, it is possible to suppress ovulation and prevent painful periods. This may be done with estrogen-progestin combinations, resulting in a very light but painless flow, or it may be done with estrogens alone. Only a doctor should make this decision and administer the pills. For at least twenty years I have used estrogens in twenty-day cycles in treating young girls with painful menstrual periods, and I have seen no complication from this treatment. In general, however, I would not advise the daily administration of pills but, rather, the twenty-day cycle method.

Q. *I have always had very heavy menstrual periods lasting up to seven or eight days. Since I have been on the pills, my flow only lasts two days. What causes this?*

A. This is due to the fact that your ovary is suppressed and the estrogen and progesterone from the ovary are no longer being secreted. The amount of estrogen and progestin in the Pill do not permit the lining of the uterus to build up to the extent that it did when you were ovulating normally. When the progestin in the Pill is a very potent one, it even produces a very thin lining of the uterus so that the flow is minimal.

Q. *Will I gain weight on the Pill?*

A. This varies with individuals. The majority of my patients, after one year on oral contraceptive agents, weigh within five pounds (above or below) of their beginning weight. Whether you gain weight or lose it or stay the same will depend in large part on your individual reaction to the Pill. Some women, so relieved of their fear of pregnancy, feel more relaxed, eat more and gain weight.

It is important to realize that some degree of weight gain may be due to water retention from the estrogen in the pill. Some women tend to gain more "water weight" than others. Such patients should utilize an oral contraceptive agent with the lower dose (.05 mg.) of estrogen. Many of my patients with this tendency toward water retention solve this problem by taking a diuretic agent at intervals during the cycle.

You should also remember that some of the progestins in the oral contraceptive agents are "anabolic." This means they tend to build muscle tissue, and they are very similar to drugs that we prescribe for weight gain. These agents are ideal for patients who are scrawny and underweight but for others, an oral contraceptive with less protein anabolic effects should be selected. The new mini-dose of Ortho-Novum-1, Norinyl-1, Noriday, and Ovral are examples of this type. (The mini-dose pills contain only 1 mg. of the progestin plus .05 mg. of estrogen compared to agents originally used which contained up to 10 mg. of progestin plus .125 mg. of estrogen.)

You should remember, also, that weight gain in general is due to excessive intake of calories. A corrective diet, low in calories, will always result in weight loss if it is adhered to.

Q. *What can I do about the nausea associated with the Pill?*

A. As I said before, I suggest that my patients take the Pill with their evening meal because I think this reduces nausea and "queasiness." The newer mini-dose pills are much less likely to cause nausea. Most women who experience nausea adjust gradually to the pill and tolerate it better as they continue to take it. In a recent study, in which half the patients took the actual birth control pill and half took a dummy pill made of sugar, it was discovered that 23 per cent of the women who took the birth control pill experienced side effects, but 17 per cent of the women who took the sugar pill felt the same effects. There is no doubt that some of the side effects are psychological.

Q. *Does the Pill lessen the natural lubricant in the vagina?*

A. No. As a matter of fact, the vagina itself does not secrete a lubricant. These secretions are derived from the glands of the cervix and from other glands, for example, Bartholin's gland, at the opening of the vagina. The estrogen in the pill actually may increase the amount of cervical secretion and is particularly valuable to women in premenopause, when their estrogen levels may be diminishing.

If additional lubrication from the glands of the cervix is desired, one of the sequential agents is preferable since the estrogen during the first fourteen to sixteen days is not opposed by a progestin.

Q. *What effect do the pills have on women with chronic cervicitis (an infection of the mouth of the uterus)?*

A. The effect is similar to that seen in pregnancy. There is no actual increase in any specific infection per se. However, since the estrogen in the Pill increases the growth of the glands that line the cervix, there may be an increased amount of discharge from the cervix and also a little increased growth of the glands on the surface of the vaginal portion of the cervix. This sometimes is known as "cervical erosion." In some cases, it is necessary to cauterize the cervix a bit more often, but since this is seen frequently in nonusers of the Pill, it is hard to interpret its increased incidence, if any.

Q. *Is it true that the Pill will cause thinning of the hair and baldness?*

A. No. But there is a similarity between the effects of some oral contraceptives and the change in the hair during pregnancy. Many women, following delivery, note that their hair seems to be falling out, but this is simply the loss of excess hair that grew during the pregnancy. If areas of baldness develop after pregnancy, it is not due to the hormonal changes, but usually to severe psychosomatic disturbances. This is the most common cause of patchy baldness or even total baldness in which the hair is lost in other portions of the body, notably the eyebrows and limbs. Focal areas of baldness (alopecia areata) are associated with the inflammation around hair shafts and are frequently of psychosomatic origin. Dr. Walter Lever of Boston, an authority on skin diseases, states that "There is no relationship between alopecia areata and the use of oral contraceptives." Most patients, in fact, complain that they notice a thickening of their hair while taking the Pill. Some patients who use the more androgenic type of oral contraceptive (those with male hormone effects) may note increased hair growth as well as acne on the face and chest. If this occurs, these patients should be shifted to a more estrogenic pill such as Enovid or possibly one of the sequential agents.

Q. *Will the Pill affect my sexual desire?*

A. In general, use of the Pill, by removing the fear of pregnancy, usually results in more pleasurable, more spontaneous, more frequent marital relations.

The complete answer to this question is probably as complex as the individual woman's attitude about sex itself. In many women, any changes in desire while on the Pill follow the same pattern as those felt during pregnancy. For some women, pregnancy is a sexually exciting time, and these women would probably react in a similar fashion to the Pill. In those women in whom sexual excitement is dulled by pregnancy, a similar diminution may be seen in relation to the Pill. These women may notice a decrease in the urge for sexual relations and a diminution in the ability to achieve orgasm. Some patients have told me that they have a marked increase in desire while taking the more androgenic pills (Ortho-Novum, Norinyl, Ovulen) and that there is a noticeable change when they shift to basically estrogenic tablets such as the sequential agents. Since male hormone itself, when administered to the female, may increase sex desire in some cases, this is clearly understandable.

Q. *Will the Pill make me promiscuous?*

A. I doubt it. Promiscuity is based upon multiple factors and with the great variety of stimuli present in the world today (alcohol, salacious literature, suggestive movies, LSD, or drugs such as marijuana which reduce inhibitions) it is difficult to state the precise impact of the Pill. In the opinion of most psychiatrists and social workers, there is no increase in promiscuous behavior in women on the Pill.

Q. *Is it true that some women become anxious while on the Pill and other are depressed?*

A. First of all, let me explain that this is not due to any variation in thyroid function. Although there are changes in the various tests which measure thyroid function, these are simply due to the effect of the estrogen in the Pill on the binding of the thyroid hormone to certain proteins. Let's take it from the beginning, however. Progesterone is a hormone which depresses the central nervous system. If given in adequate amount, it can produce drowsiness and sleep in the experimental animal. One of the very characteristic symptoms of early pregnancy is that of "a tired or drowsy feeling." Obstetricians look upon this as a good sign, since it indicates that the normal levels of progesterone are present.

A very few patients apparently have a hypersensitivity to the progestin in the Pill. And, rather amazingly, this sensitivity may result in either anxiety or depression. Each month that the patient is on the Pill, the symptoms of either one of these side effects increase. Since there are so many other stress factors present that can cause anxiety and depression, it is very difficult to assess the proportion caused by the Pill.

If symptoms persist beyond the third or fourth month, particularly symptoms of depression and lethargy, I usually discontinue the oral contraceptive and prescribe another method. Remember, there are only a few patients in this category.

Q. *Will the Pill cause migraine headaches?*

A. No, the Pill will not *cause* migraine headaches, but it may aggravate already existing migraine or the tendency toward migraine. Migraine is a very peculiar headache pattern. There are really two types, "true" migraine in which the attack follows a preliminary phase of nausea, vomiting, and various visual disturbances. The other "migraine-like" headache is due first to spasm, then dilation, of large blood vessels in the brain. "Menstrual" migraine is quite common and occurs just prior to the normal menstrual period. But this occurs when the hormonal levels of estrogen and progesterone are low. During pregnancy, that is, when hormone levels are high, migraine headaches are uncommon. Migraine attacks may occur during the period of the perimenopause, when hormonal levels are fluctuating, but a year or so after complete menopause, one finds that migraine attacks rarely occur. What does this all mean? Well, it may actually mean that the vascular changes in the brain which cause migraine are related to a rise and then a fall of estrogen and progesterone. Recent work in Sweden suggests that some patients may have their migraine attacks brought on or aggravated by estrogen, but that a constant daily dose of a pure progestin pill greatly diminishes the incidence of migraine. I have found that patients who are on "pseudopregnancy"* with high doses of estrogen and progestin develop migraine infrequently, much as in pregnancy. At the present time, therefore, I would suggest that women who have a history of migraine headaches utilize the "progestin only" method of contraception.

Q. *I heard that the Pill causes blood clots and occasionally death. Is this true?*

A. There is no doubt that some women, apparently healthy, developed blood clots in veins (thrombophlebitis) while taking the Pill. A few developed pulmonary emboli (spread of the clot to the lung) and some of those with pulmonary emboli died. But to state that this is "cause and effect," statisticians must first prove that the incidence of thrombophlebitis and pulmonary emboli is higher in users than in nonusers of the Pill. In studies published by the National Disease and Therapeutic Index and the Medical Research Council, it was determined that the incidence of thrombophlebitis was 2.2 cases per 1,000 women per year in nonpregnant

---

* "Pseudopregnancy" is a method of treatment for endometriosis in which estrogens plus progestins are taken daily—every day—not in 20- or 21-day cycles. It may be continued for one or two years.

women of childbearing age based on visits to physicians. The normal incidence of thrombophlebitis in nonpregnant women of childbearing age is *1 case per 1,000 women* per year based on hospital admissions. But in a review of six large-scale studies of 50,781 women using *oral contraceptives,* the average incidence of thrombophlebitis was only 0.55 per 1,000 women per year. This figure, 0.5/1,000, is exactly the same as that reported *during pregnancy*—but for only nine months—not twelve. A recent study published in the *British Medical Journal* indicates that while the oral contraceptives double a woman's chances of developing blood clots, being pregnant *quadruples* the chance.

An August, 1966, report of the Advisory Committee on Obstetrics and Gynecology to the Federal Food and Drug Administration states: "The most recent response on the blood relation factors to the oral contraceptives indicated no statistically significant evidence, and the data derived from mortality statistics are not adequate to confirm or refute the role of oral contraceptives in thrombophlebic disease."

I have prescribed contraceptive pills both before and after surgery I have performed for endometriosis. In over three hundred patients so treated, none has developed thrombophlebitis or pulmonary embolism. I would have suspected that the administration of an agent which caused blood clots would have caused this condition in at least a few patients. It did not. To summarize, let's accept the risk indicated by the latest British report of a sevenfold increased risk of death due to blood clots in users of the Pill over nonusers. But be fully aware of three important points: (1) the risk is extremely small, 1.5 per 100,000 in users age twenty to thirty-four and 3.9 per 100,000 in users ages thirty-five to forty-four; (2) should pregnancy occur using another method, the risk of death from all causes is 22.8 per 100,000 and 57.6 per 100,000 for the same age groups; (3) the quoted study is retrospective, that is, it is based upon women who had already developed blood clots. No controlled *prospective* study, that is, starting from scratch with matched pairs, then following these individuals for a specified period of time, has as yet been reported.

Q. *I recently read an editorial which demanded that the FDA halt sale of birth control pills in the United States. One doctor called the Pill "the most dangerous drug ever introduced for use by the healthy in respect to the lethality and major complications." Whom is the patient supposed to believe?*

A. Well, personally I would believe the statements and the statistics of the individuals who have actually been involved in using the Pill rather than the statements of those who have never used them. Dr. Louis Hellman, Chairman of the United States Food and Drug Administration's Advisory Committee on Obstetrics and Gynecology, has stated that he thinks the Pill is as safe as or safer than a diaphragm as a means of contraception. He explains it this way: "If you have 100,000 women who do not wish to become pregnant and use the pill, three may die from blood clots to the lung.

"If you have 100,000 women who do not wish to become pregnant and use a diaphragm, 10,000 *will* become pregnant. Among these 10,000 pregnant women, 3 or 4 can be expected to die as a result of the pregnancy alone."

Dr. Duncan E. Reid, Professor of Obstetrics and Gynecology at Harvard Medical School, believes that in the long run the deaths in the British study will turn out to be associated with some disease present in the women before they went on the Pill.

Dr. Hellman has also commented, "We have to evaluate the risk from use of the pill in terms of other risks that women take, such as riding in automobiles and smoking cigarettes. It's ten times more dangerous to ride in an automobile than to take contraceptive pills. And the pill is about as dangerous as smoking three cigarettes a day." The intrauterine device is not without some danger of death. About 2 of every 100,000 users will have a perforation of the uterus leading to fatal peritonitis. Dr. Hellman concluded that the benefits of the oral contraceptives so far outweigh the risks associated with their use that *they remain the preferred method of family planning.*

I think you should realize that the physician who made the statement about the Pill's being "the most dangerous drug" for use by a healthy individual has objected strenuously to its use on moral grounds even before side effects and complications were reported.

He has stated further, "The public was propagandized to the efficiency of a modality whose safety was in question while an attempt was made to upset the American people about a population explosion which didn't exist in this country." Personally, I do not believe that the American female uses the Pill because of a fear of the population crisis. She wishes only to plan the size of her family and has found other methods, including rhythm, inadequate.

Q. *I have heard that the Pill causes "strokes" and even blindness. Is there any evidence for this statement?*

A. The study in the *British Medical Journal* concerning thrombophlebitis stated that the oral contraceptives are probably *not* associated with an increased risk of heart attack but *may* enhance the chances of a stroke. Other studies concerning stroke are inconclusive and researchers agree that the hazard, if any, is small.

One prospective study comparing users and nonusers of the Pill between 1960 and 1965 showed no significant difference between the two groups. Women having severe migraine headaches, however, especially when these attacks are accompanied by some symptoms such as numbness of the hands or impaired vision, should stop the Pill and secure medical consultation. The original report of stroke association with the Pill cited only nine patients and did not claim or establish a statistical relationship between strokes, migraine, and the Pill.

I know of no instance where blindness was associated with the use of the Pill. In the original report from Johns Hopkins Hospital, eye symptoms were reported in sixty-three patients who were taking the Pill. However, the authors stated that the available data did not prove a direct relationship between the pills and the reactions cited in the report. Remember that these sixty-three patients represent the total of all referred patients to a well-known eye clinic. In my own practice during the last ten years I cannot recall one patient who had eye symptoms that necessitated discontinuing the Pill.

Another study has shown a rather high incidence of abnormalities in the eye of patients *before* they started on the Pill. If their eyes had not been carefully examined until after use of the Pill, it is quite obvious that erroneous conclusions could have been made.

Q. *If I have had hepatitis or jaundice, should I take the Pill?*

A. Women with existing liver disease should not take the Pill because of the extra work load placed on the liver by the estrogen-progestin involved, these hormones being metabolized (that is, processed) in the liver. Jaundice has been reported with some of the progestins but this is a dose-related problem and with the newer mini-doses the incidence is extremely small.

If you have had "pregnancy jaundice," it is probable that you have an inborn defect in liver metabolism and the jaundice will reccur when you take the Pill. Therefore, you should not take the Pill.

If you have had hepatitis in the past, your doctor should do the usual liver function tests to determine if your liver has returned to its normal state. If these tests are normal, there is no reason to worry about taking the Pill.

Q. *I am a diabetic and I take insulin. Can I take the Pill safely?*

A. The administration of the Pill to women who are known diabetics is not strictly prohibited, but caution should be used in prescribing these agents. It may be of more importance, although we are not sure of this, not to give the Pill to women who are in a pre-diabetic state.

There is no doubt that some change in glucose tolerance occurs in some women taking the Pill. This usually returns to normal when the Pill is discontinued. In some women it even returns to normal before the Pill is discontinued. But these changes are similar to those noted during normal pregnancy.

Most specialists who treat diabetes do not believe that the Pill will produce "true" diabetes in women who demonstrate abnormal glucose tolerance while taking the Pill. However, these specialists continue to keep these women under observation and to repeat the test at regular intervals.

There is no doubt that pregnancy poses a very serious problem for the severe diabetic. These women are limited in the number of children they can safely have. Therefore, most clinics which specialize in diabetes rely heavily on oral contraception. Dr. Priscilla White, of the Joslin Clinic in Boston, has for years given estrogen and progesterone in large doses to severe diabetic patients during pregnancy in the hope that it will improve the delivery of normal babies in these cases.

In summary, the slight risk of the Pill is preferable to the known hazards of pregnancy for women with overt diabetes.

Q. *My gynecologist told me that I have a fibroid uterus. Is it safe for me to take the Pill?*

A. I think it is *safe* for you to take the Pill, but I must make certain qualifications. First of all, it will depend to a certain extent on the size and position of the fibroid and also on the type of pill you are taking.

There is no doubt that the growth of a fibroid depends on estrogen. But remember your own ovaries may produce more estrogen each month than you get in twenty-one pills. No one claims that the Pill *causes* fibroids, but in a recent survey of specialists in obstetrics and gynecology, over half were convinced that the Pill increased the *rate of growth* of fibroids. If I decided that, because of the small size of the fibroid, and the inability of the patient to use other contraceptive measures, I wanted to prescribe the Pill, then I would select one with the lowest amount of estrogen and a progestin with a very marked antiestrogenic effect. Furthermore, I would insist that my patient return for frequent pelvic examinations, usually every three months. An even better method would be to use one of the newer agents which utilize only progestin and no estrogen. However, these are available only in centers where these agents are being tested. Or, one could treat a patient of this type with injections of Depo-Provera, a progestational compound which is not estrogenic. I have treated many women with fibroids by injections every three months—none became pregnant.

Q. *Is it true that the Pill might cause cancer of the breast or uterus?*

A. No. There is no statistically valid evidence that either the progestin or the estrogen in the Pill will *cause* cancer of any organ in the human female. As a matter of fact, there is clinical evidence to suggest that the progestin in the Pill might actually prevent the development of cancer of the lining of the uterus.

There is no doubt that the estrogen present in the Pill may aggravate an already existing cancer of the breast, and it is for this reason that physicians have insisted on breast examination every six months while the Pill is being administered. Actually, early diagnosis of breast cancer is made possible by regular, scheduled examinations. One method of accomplishing this is to insist on examination before prescribing the Pill and every six months thereafter.

Cancer of the cervix is not caused by either estrogen or progesterone (or the progestins) in the Pill. However, by insisting upon regular examinations and by doing a Pap smear at least annually, the diagnosis of very early cervical cancer may be made. Thus, cancer can be prevented! This is our ultimate goal—prevention rather than treatment. Although a woman who has already been treated for cancer of the cervix would have no need for a contraceptive (since she would have been rendered sterile by radium, x-ray, or hysterectomy), I have routinely given estrogen to these women to prevent the symptoms of menopause. This accentuates our opinion regarding the nonhormonal aspect of cervical cancer.

Q. *Is it true that women who take the Pill have an increased tendency to develop abnormal Pap smears?*

A. Of course, the answer depends on whether women who select the Pill have an increased prevalence of diseases of the cervix before they began using the Pill. I know of no evidence that the Pill, per se, changes the normal cells of the cervix and in our clinic at the Boston Hospital for Women we have not seen an increased number of pill users with abnormal Pap smears during the past ten years. Several recent studies of indigent population groups have shown a high prevalence of abnormal Pap smears and a premalignant change in the cervix called "cancer-in-situ." But remember that this is to be expected and an increased incidence of abnormal smears in users versus non-users has not been demonstrated. Cancer of the cervix occurs more commonly in women in the lower socio-economic bracket, women who have had frequent intercourse before the age of twenty, particularly in women who have had multiple sexual partners prior to that age. Cancer of the cervix is, therefore, common in prostitutes and rare in virgins. The use of a diaphragm may protect, to a certain degree, against cancer of the cervix because it prevents contact of the penis with the cervix and there is accumulating evidence that this type of cancer may be of virus origin. One might conclude that a young girl might be led to have more frequent intercourse prior to age twenty because of the availability of the Pill and therefore, at least indirectly, the Pill caused her to develop cancer. But if this same girl has a Pap smear every year, I can assure you that changes in the cervix, correctable changes, will be found before she progresses to "cancer-in-situ."

Q. *Is it true that women who have a family history of cancer of the breast should not take the Pill?*

A. Neither a straight yes nor a straight no may be given as a correct answer to this question. There has been a recent furore regarding the use of oral contraceptives in women who have a strong family history of breast cancer. There is no doubt that there is an increased incidence in women whose mothers or sisters have had this disease. For example, daughters of women with breast cancer have twenty-eight times as much chance of having breast cancer as women in the population at large. Sisters of breast cancer victims run a risk forty times as great as women in general. However, the conclusion has already been stated that there is no direct correlation between the Pill and breast cancer. As a matter of fact, the conclusions derived by the authors of the most recent paper published in the *New England Journal of Medicine* were: "The facts merely indicate that oral contraceptives have an impact on breast physiology and anatomy. They do not establish any clear association with breast cancer itself." They also conclude that "In a young, married woman with a positive family history of breast cancer, one can hardly support the *prolonged* use of contraceptive pills to avoid pregnancy, lactation and nursing." If lactation and nursing *diminish* the incidence of breast cancer, then any method of conception control would tend to *increase* the incidence simply by prevention of the physiological breast dangers associated with pregnancy.

Certainly the most important aspect regarding breast cancer in these individuals is the prevention of that disease and the only effective preventive method against widespread breast cancer is early diagnosis by palpation and possibly by x-ray.

I administer oral contraceptives to patients in whom the family history indicates mammary carcinoma, but I insist that these patients visit me frequently, because I believe it is only by early palpation of the lesion that early diagnosis and effective treatment may be accomplished.

If a close follow-up of the patient is not possible, I would not administer the Pill to patients with a family history of breast cancer.

Q. *I recently had a lump removed from my breast which the doctor said was benign. May I take the Pill?*

A. This depends on the precise diagnosis of the tissue that was removed as the "lump." If it was a benign growth known as a "fibroadenoma" I would have no reservations about giving you the Pill. Similarly, if it was the garden variety of fibrocystic disease, also known as chronic cystic mastitis, I would also administer the Pill. However, if the tissue showed excessive or unusual growth patterns which are seen prior to the development of breast cancer, I would not prescribe oral contraceptives.

Q. *I have heard that after the Pill is discontinued, the menstrual periods sometimes do not recur for a long period of time and that these women are then infertile.*

A. Physicians and clinical investigators conducting long-term trials of the pills report that: (1) oral contraceptives have *no* deleterious effect on future fertility; (2) ovulation returns promptly (usually within a month) after the pills are stopped; (3) the pregnancy rate for women discontinuing oral contraceptives is significantly higher than the rate for women discontinuing other methods of contraception, *if they have proven fertility before going on the Pill.*

Research reports have shown that 75 per cent of women who want to have babies become pregnant within three cycles after stopping the Pill and 90 per cent conceive within one year. An occasional woman does not become pregnant or even resume menstruation for months or even years afterwards. But, in most cases, these are women who have never been pregnant before. It is important to remember that 7 per cent of women will not become pregnant whether they take the Pill or not. In regard to those patients, one cannot state that the inability to become pregnant is a responsibility of the Pill. Furthermore, after having had one normal pregnancy and delivery there is no evidence at present to indicate that this "secondary infertility" is increased in women who have used the Pill.

It is important for you, and your physician, to remember that secondary amenorrhea (cessation of menstrual periods) may be caused by a variety of factors from pituitary tumors to over-activity of the adrenal gland. Therefore, if a woman does not menstruate within two or three months after discontinuing the Pill, it behooves the physician to initiate a complete investigation and search for the exact cause of lack of menstruation. In my opinion, it is poor medical practice to assume that the lack of menstruation is due to the previous use of the Pill, since a pituitary tumor may be missed and serious damage occur.

Q. *Is any treatment available for women who do not begin to menstruate within three or four months after discontinuing the Pill?*

A. Yes, the drug Clomid (clomiphene citrate) is very effective in inducing ovulation in patients with this type of lack of menstruation.

Q. *Is it a good idea to stop taking the Pill for short intervals every year or two to let the body establish a normal relationship between the pituitary and the ovary?*

A. Yes, I think that this is a good idea in certain patients. Although the Food and Drug Administration has lifted all time limits on use of the Pill, some obstetricians and gynecologists insist that their patients take an occasional breather from the Pill. In one study, it was shown that one in four physicians takes his patients off the drug within two years. Personally, I think this should be done in women in the younger age group who have not demonstrated their ability to become pregnant.

Q. *I've heard that when you go off the Pill, you are more fertile. Is this true?*

A. This is apparently true, at least in some studies, but only in women who have demonstrated their ability to become pregnant and to maintain pregnancy before taking the Pill. It is not known whether this is due to a "rebound" of pituitary hormones, or to a better development of the lining of the uterus so that implantation of the egg may occur with ease.

Q. *Do the pills affect babies born to mothers who have discontinued oral contraceptives to become pregnant?*

A. There is no report of the Pill ever having affected babies born to mothers who have terminated the oral contraceptive program. I think you are confusing the very minor deformities of the external female genitalia that were reported in some babies born to patients who took the Pill, usually in very large doses, during the first four to ten weeks of pregnancy. Some of the pills contain a progestin which is "male-like" in its potential. If this is taken in adequate amounts when the external female organs are developing in the baby, she may show enlargement of the clitoris and fusion of the labia, the external structures at the vaginal opening. This can be corrected by very minor surgery. In any event, it is not advisable to take a contraceptive pill during early pregnancy.*

Q. *Is the incidence of abortion higher in pregnancies which occur shortly after discontinuing the Pill?*

A. No. Statistical surveys of numerous groups in the United States, United Kingdom and in the prolonged Puerto Rico study do not show an increased incidence of abortion. One recent report of abnormal chromosomes in the fetus of women who aborted after stopping the Pill showed an increased number of fetuses with chromosomal abnormalities. But since the overall incidence of abortion is not increased it cannot be concluded that the Pill increases the rate at which these abnormalities occur. It is also possible that other factors might have caused the chromosomal abnormalities since even cyclamates used as a sweetener in diet drinks have been shown to have this property in the test tube and in animals.

Q. *What would happen to a woman if she took the pills as long as ten or fifteen years?*

* An exception is Provest, since the progestin in this pill is neuter.

A. No one can answer this question with certainty, although the Pill has had no harmful effect on women who have been taking it for ten consecutive years. Currently, the Food and Drug Administration has removed the curb on the length of use.

Q. *After taking the Pill regularly for six years and then stopping, how long must I wait for my periods to start?*

A. This depends, to a certain extent, on your age. If you are in your twenties or thirties, you should have a normal menstrual period within three or four months. If this does not occur I would suggest that you see your physician so that a diagnostic survey may be made to determine the cause of your lack of ovulation and menstruation. However, if you are in your mid-forties and take the Pill for four or five years, you may never have another spontaneous menstruation, since you may have entered the menopause. This would not be evident to you because the pills merely substituted the usual hormones of the ovary. If you are in this age group and do not have a menstrual period within one year, I would strongly suspect that you are now "postmenopausal."

Q. *How much research has been done on women in their early forties who are not in the menopausal stage? I have heard that the Pill affects their menopause more.*

A. A woman in her early forties should start to ovulate and menstruate within three to four months of discontinuing the Pill if the ovaries have not been depleted of their eggs. To reiterate, taking the Pill in no way affects the age at which menopause would normally occur.

In regard to the amount of research done, I would estimate that more research has been done in all aspects of this particular field than in any other concerning the effects of the Pill. Not only that, extensive research is going on at the present time to study the possible beneficial effects of the Pill (particularly its estrogen content) in the prevention of specific diseases of aging, namely, atherosclerosis (hardening of the arteries) and osteoporosis (brittleness of bones).

Q. *Does the Pill postpone the menopause?*

A. No, there is no evidence that oral contraceptives postpone— or hurry—the beginning of the menopause. Any statement that the

Pill will postpone the menopause has no basis in scientific evidence. Such a statement completely disregards the natural aging process of the ovary and the natural diminution in fertility even of patients who ovulate regularly beyond the age of forty years. Pregnancy after age fifty-six has not been reported in women of great parity (many pregnancies) who have ovulated only fifteen or sixteen times during their lifetimes. It should be remembered that the eggs are not simply stored in the ovary during the period of pill taking, but undergo a process of development and degeneration very similar to that seen during normal pregnancy.

There have been a few cases reported of women who have had a spontaneous premature menopause, say at age thirty or thirty-two, who then began to ovulate again spontaneously at age thirty-eight or thirty-nine and have become pregnant. But remember that this occurs spontaneously and is not related to the Pill.

Q. *Will the Pill disguise the arrival of the menopause?*

A. Yes. As previously mentioned, if a woman continues to take the Pill, say even until age seventy-five, she will continue to have withdrawal bleeding episodes each month. However, these are not "menstrual flows," because menstruation implies previous ovulation. This woman would have stopped ovulating and menstruating at the normal age, roughly fifty or fifty-two, but the bleeding episodes occur regularly if the Pill is continued. Furthermore, she will not experience any of the severe reactions caused by changes in blood vessels such as hot flashes, flushes, and excessive perspiration, because adequate estrogen is provided during this period of time by the Pill.

Q. *Is the Pill that is prescribed for the treatment of menopause the same as the oral contraceptives?*

A. Not necessarily. Most physicians use an estrogen alone after a woman has passed the menopausal period of life. The administration of estrogens *alone* will relieve the symptoms associated with the menopause, but will not, if given correctly, result in withdrawal bleeding. Most gynecologists, and I agree with this concept, use the contraceptive pill if the woman is in the pre-menopausal period. This affords her the benefit of conception control (which oral estrogen alone does not do), gives her regular withdrawal bleeding, prevents the development of menopausal symptoms and, even further, prevents the development of over-growth of the lining of the uterus which might become cancerous.

Q. *Many doctors have advised against the use of the Pill. Isn't this enough reason for patients to be suspicious of its possible effects?*

In my opinion there is no reason why any doctor should advise against the use of the Pill except for specific medical reasons—a few of which we've discussed. Since the medication was first tested twelve years ago, numerous articles have appeared which cite a few case reports of practically every disorder or disease that occurs spontaneously in women ages fifteen to forty-five. I know of no article which *proves* a cause-and-effect relationship. On the contrary, many articles have appeared which confirm the findings of the original study.

Some doctors advise against use of the Pill on moral or theological grounds. This is an acceptable reason, but not a medical one.

Doctors are free to follow their own judgment, and where there is freedom of choice, different decisions will always be made. In one committee studying the effects of the Pill on blood clots and their method of spread, the Pill was judged *not* to be a specific cause by a vote of 28–2. The two physicians who did not approve did so not because of evidence that the Pill was harmful, but rather because of their reservations about the specific wording of the conclusions of the committee. Even the conclusions of the *British Medical Journal* report of April, 1968, did not favor discontinuation of the Pill despite an apparent increased risk of blood clots in users.

The various study committees that have been appointed by the American Medical Association and the Federal Food and Drug Administration are made up of respected obstetricians and gynecologists, biochemists, pathologists, and statisticians. Most physicians throughout the United States are willing to accept the conclusions reached by these eminent authorities.

Glossary

Abortifacient—an agent that produces abortion.
Amenorrhea—lack of menstrual periods.
Anabolic—capable of building tissue, e.g., muscle.
Androgens—male hormones, the most potent being testosterone.
Androstenedione—a male hormone that is converted to female hormone in the ovary.

Biopsy—procedure to obtain a sample of tissue, usually from the cervix or womb lining.
Breakthrough bleeding—bleeding *while taking* the pills.

Carcinogen—an agent that causes cancer.
Climacteric—a "critical" period of life, e.g., the menopause in the female.
Combination pills—oral contraceptives containing both estrogen and a progestin.
Corpus luteum—literally "yellow body"; the site of rupture of the follicle on the ovary from which the egg is released.
Curettage—scraping of the lining of the womb, usually for diagnostic purposes.

D. & C.—*Dilatation* of the cervix (mouth of the womb) and *Curettage* (scraping) of the lining of the womb.

Diuretic—an agent that increases the output of urine, usually for the relief of bloating or swelling.

Dysmenorrhea—painful menstrual periods.

Edema—bloating or swelling of body tissues.

Embolism—obstruction of a blood vessel (as in the lungs).

Endometriosis—fragments of tissue lining the womb (endometrium) which spread to the pelvic organs via the Fallopian tubes—then function each month as miniature wombs.

Endometrium—lining of the womb (uterus) which is cast off each month in the menstrual flow.

Estradiol—one of the estrogens made by the ovary; also used in the Pill as ethinyl estradiol.

Estrogen—a term for all substances that produce estrus (heat) in female animals; an all-inclusive term for the hormones made by the ovarian follicle before ovulation.

Estrone—one of many estrogenic hormones; a component of the preparation Premarin.

Fallopian tubes—paired ducts attached to the womb—they transport the egg from the ovary to the womb.

"Femininity index"—an estimate of estrogen activity based on a count of various types of cells from the vagina.

Fibroid—a benign tumor of the womb made up of muscle and fibrous tissue.

Follicle—a blister on the ovary which contains the egg and which, during its development, secretes estrogen.

FSH—"Follicle Stimulating Hormone"—a pituitary hormone that stimulates the follicle to grow.

Hyperplasia—excessive growth, usually referring to the lining of the womb.

Hypothalamus—an area of the brain that regulates function of the pituitary gland.

Hysterectomy—removal of the womb.

Implant—a plastic material containing hormones (synthetic progestins) inserted under the skin to suppress ovulation or prevent implantation of the fertilized egg.

Implantation—the process by which the fertilized ovum imbeds in the lining of the womb.

In situ—a term signifying a state of premalignant change before cancer develops.

IUD—a plastic intrauterine device inserted into the womb to prevent conception.

LH—"Luteinizing Hormone"—a pituitary hormone that produces release of the egg from the follicle, i.e., ovulation.

Mastitis—a benign condition of the breast characterized by a lumpy or nodular consistency.

Osteoporosis—increased porosity or thinning of bones, usually referring to the vertebrae.

Ovulation—release of the egg from the follicle on the ovary.

Pap test or smear—Papanicolaou smear—a test for cancer of the cervix or uterus obtained by aspirating or scraping cells from the mouth of the womb.

Peritoneum—lining of the body cavity.

Polyp—a fleshy tumor, usually benign, on the cervix or in the womb.

Postmenopausal—period of a woman's life after menstruation ceases, usually after age fifty.

Premalignant—a stage preceding the development of cancer.

Premenopausal—period of a woman's life when menstruation becomes scanty or less frequent, usually between ages 45 and 50.

Progesterone—the hormone secreted by the corpus luteum after ovulation that prepares the lining of the womb for implantation of the fertilized egg.

Progestin—a synthetic progesterone used in combination with estrogen in the Pill.

Pseudopregnancy—uninterrupted use of a pill containing an estrogen and progestin, producing lack of menstruation and many symptoms of pregnancy.

Sequential pills—oral contraceptives in which a sequence of sixteen estrogen pills are followed by five estrogen-plus-progestin pills.

Testosterone—the most potent male hormone, made in the testis of the male but also the ovary of the female.

Thromboembolism—process of clot (thrombus) breaking loose and lodging and obstructing a blood vessel.

Thrombophlebitis—a clot (thrombus) in a vein with associated inflammation.

Trichomonas infections—a common vaginal infection caused by a protozoan, *trichomonas vaginalis.*

Tubal ligation—tying off the Fallopian tubes for sterilization.

Vaginitis—infection or inflammation of the vagina.

Vas deferens—the duct by which sperm travel from the testes to the ejaculatory apparatus and penis.

Vaso-motor symptoms—hot flashes, sweats, skin-tingling, blushing—caused by changes in blood-vessel caliber associated with the climacteric.

Withdrawal flow—the bleeding that occurs after the pills are stopped—caused by the breakdown of the womb lining after "withdrawal" of estrogen and progestin support.

Yeast infections—thick, white, flaky discharges in the vagina, similar to infant "thrush," due to a fungus, *monilia albicans.*

Zygote—the individual produced by the fusion of egg and sperm cells.

References

1. Kistner, R. W. "Therapeutic Application of Progestational Compounds in Gynecology." In *Advances in Obstetrics and Gynecology*, edited by S. L. Marcus and C. C. Marcus. Baltimore: The Williams and Wilkins Co., 1967.

2. Kistner, R. W. "Histological Effects of Progestins on Hyperplasia and Carcinoma in Situ of the Endometrium." *Cancer* (1959), 18:1563

3. Kistner, R. W. "Feminine Forever? An Evaluation of Therapy During Menopause." *Medical Science* (1967), 18:42.

4. Kistner, R. W. "Hormonal Treatment of Endometriosis," *Clin. Obst. & Gynec.* (1966), 9:3.

5a. Kistner, R. W. *Idem*, Ref. 1.

5b. Shearman, R. P., "Hormonal Treatment of Habitual Abortion." In *Progress in Infertility*, edited by S. J. Behrman and R. W. Kistler. Boston: Little, Brown and Company, 1968.

6. Younge, P. A. "Cancer of the Uterine Cervix — A Preventable Disease." *Obst. & Gynec.* (1957), 10:469.

7. Kistner, R. W., Steiner, G. J., and Craig, J. M. "Histological Effect of Progestins on Hyperplasia and Carcinoma in Situ of the Endometrium—Further Observations." *Metabolism* (1965), 14: 356.

8. Kistner, R. W. and Griffiths, C. T. "Use of Progestational Agents in the Management of Metastatic Carcinoma of the Endometrium." *Clin. Obst. & Gynec.* (1968), 11:439.

9. Kistner, R. W. "The Use of Progestational Agents in Obstetrics and Gynecology." *Clin. Obst. & Gynec.* (1960), 3:1047.

10. Connell, E. B., and Kelman, C. D. "Ophthalmologic Findings with Oral Contraceptives." *Obst. & Gynec.*, Vol. 32 (1968), 456.

11. Inman, W. H. W., and Vessey, M. P. "Investigation of Deaths from Pulmonary, Coronary, and Cerebral Thrombosis and Embolism in Women of Child-bearing Age." *British Medical Journal* (1968), 2:193.

12. Vessey, M. P., and Doll, R. "Investigation of Relation Between Use of Oral Contraceptives and Thromboembolic Disease." *British Medical Journal* (1968), 2:199.

13. Drill, V. A., and Calhoun, D. W. "Oral Contraceptives and Thromboembolic Disease." *Journal of the American Medical Assn.* (1968), 206:77.

14. Kourides, I. "Freedom of Birth: Methods of Population Control Today." *Medical Science* (August, 1967), pp. 25–31.

15. Calderone, M. S. *Manual of Contraceptive Practice.* Baltimore: The Williams and Wilkins Co., 1964.

16. Kistner, R. W. *Principles and Practice of Gynecology.* Chicago: Year Book Medical Publishers, 1964.

17. Tietze, C. "Fifth Progress Report of the Cooperative Statistical Program for the Evaluation of Intra-Uterine Contraceptive Devices."

18. Sodhy, L. S. "Population Control in the Malaysian Peninsula." *Clinical Trials Journal* (London) (January, 1968).

19. Pincus, G. "Control of Conception by Hormonal Steroids." *Science,* Vol. 153 (1967), 493–500.

20. Technical Bulletin. American College of Obstetricians and Gynecologists. No. 10 (September, 1968).

21. Maisel, A. Q. *The Hormone Quest.* New York: Random House, 1965.

22. Rocamora, H., Garcia, C. R., and Pincus, G. "Long Term Effects of Oral Contraceptives." Presented at the Fifth Annual Meeting of the American Association of Planned Parenthood Physicians, Atlanta, Georgia, April 3, 1967.

23. Aldridge, L. "Why They Quit the Pill." *McCall's* (November, 1968).

24. Ryder, N. B., and Westoff, C. F. "Use of Contraception in the United States, 1965." *Science* (September, 1966), 153:1199.
25. Garcia, C. R. "Ten Years' Evaluation of Human Pharmacology of the Oral Contraceptives." *Clinical Trials Journal* (Special Issue; January, 1968), 5:17.
26. Lake, A. "Analysis of ACOG Questionnaire." *McCall's* (November, 1967).
27. Nevin, R. *British Medical Journal* (1965), 1:1586.
28. Illis, C. *British Medical Journal* (1965), 2:1164.
29. Larsson-Cohn, P. *J.A.M.A.* (1965), 193:422.
30. Kleiner, G. S. "Studies of Hepatic Excretory Function." *New England Journal of Medicine* (1965), 273:420.
31. Spellacy, W. N., and Carlson, K. L. *American Journal of Obstetrics and Gynecology* (1966), 95:474.
32. Wallach, S., and Henneman, P. H. "Prolonged Estrogen Therapy in Postmenopausal Women." *J.A.M.A.* (1959), 171:1637.
33. *New Drugs Evaluated by the A.M.A. Council on Drugs.* Chicago, 1967, p. 377.
34. Gusberg, S. B., and Kaplan, A. L. "Precursors of Corpus Cancer." *American Journal of Obstetrics and Gynecology* (1963), 87:662.
35. Hertig, A. T., and Sommers, S. C. "Genesis of Endometrial Carcinoma." *Cancer* (1949), 2:946.
36. Naismith, G. "Common Sense and the Femininity Pill." *Reader's Digest* (September, 1966).
37. Kaufman, S. A. *The Ageless Woman: Menopause, Hormones and the Quest for Youth.* Englewood Cliffs, N.J.: Prentice-Hall, 1967.
38. Blum, S. "The Pill." *Redbook* (January, 1966).
39. Neubardt, S. *A Concept of Contraception.* New York: Trident, 1967.
40. Rice-Wray, E., *et al. British Medical Journal,* 1964, 2:1094; *Fertility and Sterility,* 1963, 14:402.
41. Shiloh, A. Paper presented before the American Association for the Advancement of Science, New York City, 1967.
42. Berland, T. "What the Pill Is Doing to Husbands." *Cosmopolitan* (December, 1966).
43. Osterman, R., and Arnold, M. *The Pill and Its Impact.* A Newsbook —*The National Observer.* Silver Spring, Maryland, 1967.
44. Masters, W., and Johnson, V. *Human Sexual Response.* Boston: Little, Brown and Company, 1966.
45. Connell, E. B. *Ob-Gyn News,* Vol. 3: No. 15 (August 1, 1968).

46. Tyler, E. Paper presented at A.M.A. meeting, June, 1968.
47. Bald, W. *Women's News Service*, August, 1968.
48. Rock, J. *The Time Has Come*. New York: Alfred A. Knopf, 1963.
49. Spencer, S. M. "The Birth Control Revolution." *Saturday Evening Post* (January 15, 1966).
50. Cunneen, S. *Sex: Female; Religion: Catholic*. New York: Holt, Rinehart and Winston, 1968.
51. Gallup Poll, American Institute of Public Opinion, 1968.
52. *U.S. News and World Report* (November 6, 1967).
53. Reston, J. *New York Times* News Service.
54. Lelyveld, J. Special to *New York Times* (August 16, 1968).
55. Ketchel, M. *Perspectives in Biology and Medicine*. 1968. 11:687.
56. Grant, M. "Family Planning in the Nation's Capital." *American Journal of Public Health* (1967).
57. Eliot, J. "The Development of Family Planning Services by State and Local Health Departments in the U.S." *American Journal of Public Health* (1967).
58. Subcommittee on Employment, Manpower, and Poverty, Committee on Labor and Public Welfare, U.S. Senate, *Family Planning Program*. Washington, 1966.
59. Subcommittee on Foreign Aid Expenditures, Committee on Government Operations, U.S. Senate, *Population Crisis, Appendix, Part 4*. Washington, D.C.

Index

cervical, 8–9, 124–25, 299–300
death rates from, 128
of endometrium, 9–10, 120–25, 183
fear of, 201
in situ, defined, 309
regular menstruation preventing, 146
studies on incidence of, 114–15
See also Breast cancer
Carcinogens, defined, 307
Carrington, Elsie R., 240
Catholic church
attitude to pill of, 192, 251–53
dissidence in, 257–58
"Of Human Life" issued by, 258–63
view of procreation of, 250–51
See also Catholics
Catholic Rhythm Committee (Boston), 268
Catholics
American Bishops' pastoral letter (1968) and, 262–63
controversies among, 253–54
Paul VI criticized by, 255–56
position on birth control of, 256–58
psychological effects of pills among, 199
reactions to "Of Human Life," 259–62
Cerebral thrombosis, 127
Cervicitis, 290
Cervix
cancer of, 8–9, 124–25, 299–300
eversion of, 107
painful menstrual periods and "closed" state of, 146–47

survival of sperm in, 21
Chang, Min-Chueh, 39
Chastity, 235
Chile, 220, 269–70
Coale, Ansley J., 268
Cobb, John C., 226
Cohen, Wilbur J., 277
Coitus interruptus, 25, 32
Colton, Frank, 43, 44
Combination pills
composition of, 50, 307
varieties of, 282
See also specific brands of combination pills
Competition in sexual relations, 205
Conception, process of, 21–23, 161, 247
Condoms
availability of, 244
disadvantages of, 24
effectiveness of, 32
protection from venereal diseases by, 238
quality of Russian, 272–73
Conn, Jerome, 101
Connell, Elizabeth, 13–14, 111, 217–18
Contraceptives; *see specific types of contraceptives*
Corpus luteum, 307
Cortisone, 19
C-Quens
action of, 287
composition of, 51, 58–59
Crossen, William J., 47
Cunneen, Sally, 257
Curettage, 307
Curran, Rev. Charles E., 263
Currie, Lauchlin, 279

reactions to postponement of families, 208

sexual regression of, 209

wives' sexual aggressiveness and, 204–205, 207

Hyperemesis gravidarum, 68–69

Hyperplasia
defined, 40, 121, 308
effects of pill on, 123
prevention of, 59

Hypothalamus, 34–35, 308

Hysterectomy, 8
defined, 308
reduced incidence of, 11
side effects of IUDs and, 29

Immunization, 231–33

Implants
defined, 309
difficulties with, 223
research on, 221–22

Implantation
defined, 309
endometrium as site of, 23; *see also* Endometrium
IUDs preventing, 29, 348–49

Impotence
causes of, 205–206

Income levels
cervical cancer and low, xvi
fertility rates and, 275–76

India
birth control in, 271–72
IUDs used in, 31
population growth in, 270–71

Infections
pelvic, 29
yeast, 310; *see also* Monilia
See also specific infections

Infertility, 153–54

abortions and, 23

after use of pill, 86

determining, 85

drug induced, 275

endometriosis and, 5, 45–46

endometrium and, 6–7

hormonal deficiency and, 6–7

Rock's experiments with, 153

spermicidal antibodies and, 232

treatment of, 41–42, 86–87, 154

See also Fertility

Inman, William H., 126–27, 273

International Planned Parenthood Federation, 243

Intrauterine devices (IUDs), 27–32
as abortifacients, 29
deaths caused by, 295
described, 309
disadvantages of, 30
effectiveness of, 32
endometrium as site of, 23;
everyday pills compared with, 218
generalizations on, 27
ideal time for insertion of, 28
implantation of ovum prevented by, 248–49
improvement of, 212, 227–28
in India, 271
in Russia, 272–73

IUDs; *see* Intrauterine devices

Japan, 246

Jaundice, 297
development of, 96
during pregnancy, 98
incidence of, 97

Jones, Howard, 132

Teenagers (*cont.*)
  venereal diseases among, 237–38
Tension
  premenstrual, 148–51, 223
  sperm production and, 206
Testosterone
  endometriosis treated with, 46
  production of, 310
Thyroid
  during menopause, 162
  effects of pill on, 38
Thromboembolism, 14–15, 130–31, 310
Thrombophlebitis
  defined, 293, 310
  incidence of, 130, 293–94
Tietze, Christopher, 29
Trichomonas
  described, 106, 310
  treatment of, 107
Tubal ligation, 229, 310
Tuberculosis, 72
Tumors, 112; *see also* Fibroid Tumors
Tydings, Joseph B., 277
Tyler, Edward, 220–21

Underdeveloped countries
  as market for IUDs, 30–31
  obstacles to development of, 279
United States
  average age of onset of menstruation in, 142
  average menopausal age in, 160
  birth rate in, 264–65
  family planning assistance provided by, 276–77
  fertility rate in, 275–76
  help provided teenagers in, 239
  illegitimate births in (1948–61), 238
  indications of osteoporosis among women in, 171
  number of pill users in, 235
  population density in, 268
  projected population of (1970), 265, 269
  venereal diseases in, 237–38
  youth fetish in, 161
United States Census Bureau, 237
Uterus
  effects of estrogen on lining of, xiv, 40
  growth of, 6
  IUDs and rupture of, 29
  size of, 21

Vaccines, 231–33
  experiments with, 232
  See also Long-acting injections
Vagina
  atrophy of, 181
  during menopause, 166–67
  secretions of, 290
Vaginal creams, 26
Vaginal discharges, 104–108
  treatment of, 105–107
  types of, 105
Vaginal foams, 26
Vaginitis, 310
Van Emde Boas, D. V., 243
Van Wagenen, Gertrude, 224, 225
Varicose veins, 17, 133
Vas deferens
  described, 310

BOOKS BY ROBERT W. KISTNER, M.D.

Principles and Practice of Gynecology.
654 pp. Chicago: Year Book Medical Publishers, 1964.
Progress in Infertility.
1033 pp. With S. J. Behrman. Boston: Little, Brown & Company, 1968.
The Progestins in Obstetrics and Gynecology.
110 pp. Chicago: Year Book Medical Publishers. On Press.
Practical Gynecologic Endocrinology.
220 pp. New York: Paul Hoeber Co., division of Harper & Row.
On Press.
Over 130 publications in medical literature.
Listed in *Who's Who in the East* and *Who's Who in Science* as the
originator of pseudopregnancy for the treatment of endometriosis
—also as one of the original investigators in the use of
Clomid for induction of ovulation.